Living with Dementia Reconsidered

Reconsidering Dementia Series Editors: Dr Keith Oliver and Professor Dawn Brooker MBE

Other titles in this series:
Dementia and Psychotherapy Reconsidered
Richard Cheston

Education and Training in Dementia Care: A Person-Centred Approach
Claire Surr, Sarah Jane Smith and Isabelle Latham

Dementia and Ethics Reconsidered
Julian C. Hughes

Leisure and Everyday Life with Dementia
Karen Gray, Christopher Russell and Jane Twigg (eds)

Reconsidering Neighbourhoods and Living with Dementia: Spaces, Places and People
John Keady (ed.)

Talking with Dementia Reconsidered
Keith Oliver, Reinhard Guss and Ruth Bartlett

Young Onset Dementia Reconsidered: A Solution-Focused Approach
Jan Oyebode and George Rook (eds)

Living with Dementia Reconsidered

Linda Clare, Catherine Charlwood, Catherine Quinn and Christina Victor (eds)

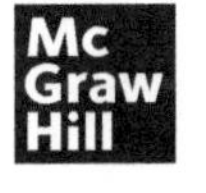

Open University Press

Open University Press
McGraw Hill
Unit 4
Foundation Park
Roxborough Way
Maidenhead
SL6 3UD

email: emea_uk_ireland@mheducation.com
world wide web: www.mheducation.co.uk

Executive Editor: Sam Crowe
Editorial Assistant: Hannah Church
Content Product Manager: Graham Jones
Cover Artwork: Jacqui Bingham and Julia Burton
Logo Design: Julia Heron
Cover Design: Adam Renvoize

A catalogue record of this book is available from the British Library

ISBN-13: 9780335252510
ISBN-10: 0335252516
eISBN-13: 9780335252527

Typeset by Transforma Pvt. Ltd., Chennai, India

O10264   ACL   2025

Praise Page

"Overall, this is an excellent resource for people studying and working in the field of dementia from a variety of disciplines. This is a book that makes a step-change in our knowledge and thinking on dementia and how living well with dementia might be defined. In particular to be commended is the strong aspect of voice from people living with dementia that found throughout. Hence the book brings together academic insight with lived experience seamlessly in adding new ways of thinking about dementia."

Professor Charles Musselwhite, Head of Psychology,
Aberystwyth University, UK

"Living with Dementia Reconsidered teaches us about what it means to live well with dementia and also how it can be supported, truly inspiring. This book provides an easy-to-understand account of authentic Patient and Public Involvement and Engagement, illuminating how the evidence can be meaningful and impactful through PPIE. The commitment and passion come through each chapter. The book is based on a longitudinal cohort study of those with lived and living experience, which would not have been possible without strong leadership and teamwork of those involved. Most of all, the book offers hope for living well with dementia."

Professor Yun-Hee Jeon, Professor of Healthy Ageing,
The University of Sydney, Australia

"For more than a decade, the IDEAL project, led by Professor Linda Clare, has been adding to our knowledge and understanding of what helps people living with dementia experience better well-being and quality of life, resulting in numerous publications in leading academic journals. IDEAL was breathtaking in scope and ground-breaking in its methods, its involvement of people living with dementia throughout the research process and its creative approaches to dissemination. This welcome volume draws together and distils the key findings and implications of the study, with remarkable clarity, accessible to all with an interest in dementia and its impact."

Bob Woods, Emeritus Professor of Clinical Psychology of Older People,
Bangor University, UK

"This book masterfully consolidates the invaluable insights from the IDEAL programme. The final chapter, with its compelling manifesto,

challenges us all to do better to improve the lives of those affected by dementia. The book is a beacon of hope and inspiration for practitioners, researchers, and policy-makers alike."

Professor Emma Wolverson, Professor of Ageing and Dementia,
University of West London / Research Lead, Dementia UK

The artwork on the book cover was created by two members of the ALWAYs group: Jacqui Bingham and Julia Burton. They collaborated on this untitled piece at a distance. They shared the following background: '*We had the idea of leaves, and we were aware we needed something which would fit on the cover, was not too detailed, and was fairly bold. We were very busy sending drawings and ideas to each other! We were also inspired by neurographic art. Neurographic art is spontaneous doodling on a theme. It brings the inside feelings and thoughts out in the art*'.

Contents

List of figures, tables, boxes, and photographs

Figures

Table

Boxes

Photographs

About the editors

Linda Clare is Professor of Clinical Psychology of Ageing and Dementia at the University of Exeter Medical School, UK. She directs the National Institute for Health and Care Research (NIHR) Policy Research Unit in Dementia and Neurodegeneration, University of Exeter and serves as dementia theme lead for the NIHR Applied Research Collaboration South-West Peninsula. Since her training in clinical psychology and neuropsychology, Linda has focused on conducting research that could improve the experiences of people who are living with dementia and their families. She has a strong interest in the potential of rehabilitation to empower people with dementia and has pioneered the application of cognitive rehabilitation approaches for people with early-stage Alzheimer's disease through the GREAT research programme. She was Chief Investigator for the IDEAL cohort study of people with dementia and carers, an Alzheimer's Society Centre of Excellence, which explored what makes it possible to experience a good quality of life with the condition and provides the basis for this book.

Catherine Charlwood was the Research Translation and Impact Manager on the IDEAL programme from 2021, and now works as Stakeholder Engagement and Impact Manager for the NIHR Policy Research Unit in Dementia and Neurodegeneration, University of Exeter. Her doctorate in literature was interdisciplinary with experimental psychology and focused on memory and poetry. She has previously published on such topics as ageing in the novels of Kazuo Ishiguro. A former schoolteacher, Catherine is particularly interested in using creative methods to engage different stakeholders. During IDEAL, she was fortunate to work closely with the ALWAYs group to co-produce resources like the Living with Dementia Toolkit.

Catherine Quinn is Associate Professor at the Centre for Applied Dementia Studies at the University of Bradford. She leads a module on post-diagnostic support and living well with dementia on the MSc in Advanced Dementia Studies. Catherine's research focuses on improving the quality of life of people living with dementia and their carers. She is currently Co-Principal Investigator of an NIHR-funded project, DYNAMIC, which focuses on improving social care planning and provision for people with young onset dementia and their families. Catherine is the Bradford University Healthy Ageing Theme Lead for the Wolfson Centre for Applied Health Research. She is a collaborator in the NIHR Policy Research Unit in Dementia and Neurodegeneration, University of Exeter and a member of the Older People's theme of the NIHR Applied Research Collaboration (ARC) Yorkshire & Humber.

Christina Victor is Professor of Gerontology and Public Health in the College of Health, Medicine and Life Sciences at Brunel University London, Associate PVC for Research Culture and Governance, and Director of the University's Institute of Health, Medicine and Environments. Christina started her academic career as a geographer with a particular interest in the spatial distribution of health and illness and access to, and provision of, health and social care. Her current research focuses on ageing and later life, with specialist interests in wellbeing, loneliness and social isolation, physical activity and exercise, care and caring, and growing old amongst minority communities. In 2017 Christina was awarded the Lifetime Achievement award of the British Society of Gerontology.

About the contributors

ALWAYs group members, The ALWAYs (Action on Living Well: Asking You) group of people living with dementia and carers contributed throughout IDEAL and co-produced outputs. Members are referred to in the text by their given names.

Catherine Charlwood PhD, IDEAL Research Translation and Impact Manager
Stakeholder Engagement and Impact Manager, NIHR Policy Research Unit in Dementia and Neurodegeneration, University of Exeter (DeNPRU Exeter), University of Exeter Medical School, Exeter, UK

Linda Clare PhD ScD, IDEAL Chief Investigator
Professor of Clinical Psychology of Ageing and Dementia, University of Exeter Medical School, Director, NIHR Policy Research Unit in Dementia and Neurodegeneration, University of Exeter (DeNPRU Exeter), and dementia theme lead, NIHR Applied Research Collaboration South-West Peninsula, Exeter, UK

Hayley Hogan MSc, IDEAL Funder Liaison
Head of Evidence and Impact, Alzheimer's Society, London, UK

Rachael Litherland MSc, IDEAL PPIE Lead
Co-Director, Innovations in Dementia, Exeter, UK

Anthony Martyr PhD, IDEAL Researcher Co-investigator
Senior Research Fellow, University of Exeter Medical School, Exeter, UK

Claire Pentecost PhD, IDEAL Programme Manager
Senior Research Fellow, University of Exeter Medical School, Exeter, UK

Catherine Quinn PhD, IDEAL Co-investigator
Associate Professor, Centre for Applied Dementia Studies, University of Bradford, Bradford, UK

Serena Sabatini PhD, IDEAL Research Associate
La Caixa Postdoctoral Research Fellow, Institute of Neurosciences, University of Barcelona, Barcelona, Spain

Sally Stapley PhD, IDEAL Research Associate
Research Fellow, Hertfordshire Business School, University of Hertfordshire, Hatfield, UK

Jeanette Thom PhD, IDEAL Co-investigator
Professor of Exercise Physiology, University of Sydney, Sydney, NSW, Australia

Christina Victor PhD, IDEAL Co-investigator
Professor of Gerontology and Public Health, Brunel University London

The Reconsidering Dementia Series

The dementia field has developed rapidly in its scope and practice over the past 25 years. Many thousands of people are newly diagnosed each year. Worldwide, the trend is that people are being diagnosed at much earlier stages. In addition, families and friends increasingly provide support to those affected by dementia over a prolonged period. Many people, both those diagnosed with dementia and those who support them, have an appetite to understand their condition. Care professionals and civic society also need an in-depth and nuanced understanding of how to support people living with dementia within their communities over the long term. The *Reconsidering Dementia* book series sets out to address this need. It takes its inspiration from the late Professor Tom Kitwood's seminal text *Dementia Reconsidered* published in 1997, which, at the time, revolutionised how dementia care was conceptualised.

The book series is jointly commissioned and edited by Professor Dawn Brooker MBE and by Dr Keith Oliver. Dawn has been active in the field of dementia care since the 1980s as a clinician and an academic. She draws on her experience and international networks to bring together a series of books on the most pertinent issues in the field. Keith is one of the foremost international advocates for those living with dementia. He also brings an insightful perspective of his own and others' experience of what it means to live with dementia gained since his diagnosis of Alzheimer's Disease in 2010.

Dawn and Keith have been professional colleagues for many years. They worked together on the second edition of Kitwood's book entitled *Dementia Reconsidered, Revisited: The Person Still Comes First*. This 2019 publication was a reprint of the original text by Tom Kitwood alongside contemporary commentaries for each chapter written by current experts. Many topics in the field of dementia care, however, were simply unheard of in Kitwood's lifetime. When Open University Press approached Dawn and Keith with the idea of developing a book series dedicated to dementia, they were very pleased to accept. The subsequent titles in this series are cutting-edge scholarly texts that challenge and engage readers to think deeply. They draw on theoretical understandings, contemporary research and experience to critically reflect on their topic in great depth.

This does not mean, however, that they are not applicable to improving the care and support of those affected by dementia. As well as the scholarly text, all books have a 'So what?' thread that unpacks what this means for people living with dementia, their families, people working in dementia care, policy-makers, professionals, community activists and so on. Too many books either focus on an academic audience OR a practitioner audience OR a student audience OR a lived experience audience. In this series, the aim is to try to address these perspectives in the round. The *Reconsidering Dementia* book series brings together the perspectives of professional practice, scholarship and the lived experience as they pertain to the key topics in the field of dementia studies. All the books aim to help us to think afresh, to reconsider our standpoint and to ultimately improve the experience of those affected by dementia for years to come.

Preface

The *Reconsidering Dementia* book series is inspired by the work of the late Professor Tom Kitwood. When Tom sent his seminal paper 'Brain, mind and dementia: with particular reference to Alzheimer's disease' to the learned journal *Ageing and Society* in 1989, the paper was considered so controversial that it was very nearly rejected outright. The basis of the controversy was that Kitwood challenged what he called the 'standard paradigm' in which dementia was conceptualised as the death that left the body behind. Through a carefully worked-through set of theoretical arguments drawing on philosophy, psychology, sociology, and neurology, he demonstrated the benefit of seeing the whole person and continuing to support personhood even though cognitive decline could be extreme. A series of papers followed written by Tom and his co-authors and this formed the basis for the book *Dementia Reconsidered* from which this series takes its name.

Given the era in which it was written, and the fact that the prevailing narrative around dementia at that time was living death, it is not surprising that the subjective experience of living with dementia was hardly touched upon in any great depth in Kitwood's writing. The importance of the subjective experience and maintaining personhood was sketched out but the richness, the light and shade, the nuance and complexity was absent. Of all the books in the *Reconsidering Dementia* series, *Living with Dementia Reconsidered* addresses this omission directly. It illuminates the colour and depth of people's experiences of living with and supporting people living with dementia over the longer term. As Linda Clare writes in her opening chapter: 'We need not just to think about dementia, but to rethink the experience of living with dementia'.

The IDEAL research programme, on which this book is based, paints in the detail about how people's lives develop with dementia. The title of the research programme IDEAL stands for 'Improving the experience of Dementia and Enhancing Active Life'. It was a major UK longitudinal programme that ran for almost 12 years and drew on the experiences of a very wide range of people affected by dementia. A particular strength of IDEAL was the participation of the ALWAYs group, drawing together a group of people living with dementia and unpaid carers. This group called themselves 'Action on Living Well: Asking You', which was shortened to ALWAYs. They were involved in the IDEAL programme from the get-go and this engagement has continued throughout the writing of this book.

This book teaches us about the importance of hope, of physical and emotional well-being, the importance of relationships, and the important influences of the context in which people live their lives. All these things work together to shape the experience of living with dementia. In addition to describing the experience of dementia, however, this book also provides the hope that the quality of people's lives can be enhanced. In its pages, we learn about the wide range of things that can make a difference to living well with dementia.

The IDEAL programme led to many papers in learned journals which have been read and cited by scholars from all over the world. The beauty of bringing the whole project together in book form, however, is that the sum of the overall research tells us much more than the parts that are written up in journal papers. Journal papers only focus on a specific aspect of the programme rather than the whole. A number of books in the *Reconsidering Dementia* series have enabled large-scale research projects to report in this way. As series editors, we were thrilled to receive the proposal for a book based on the IDEAL programme. We both knew the quality of the research from our different perspectives. Even so, the finished book has surpassed our expectations. We hope you enjoy its riches here as much as we did.

Series Editors: Dawn Brooker and Keith Oliver

Additional thoughts from Keith Oliver

I never expected that my first connection with the IDEAL project at Alzheimer's Society head office on a wet, cool London day on 1 April 2014 would result in an involvement which took me to places I would never have believed I would visit; to hear things I was moved by; to contribute in ways I never knew I could achieve; and to be inspired in ways that no other project could, nor do I expect will do, in the future. This latest contribution to the *Dementia Reconsidered* book series is a significant and important addition to the collection, as it truly shows the impact a major research project can have on the lives of those affected by dementia alongside providing the necessary resonance between professionals and service users.

It has been a genuine privilege and honour to serve on the Project Advisory Group since day one and likewise as a member of the renowned ALWAYs group – the latter really should be a role model for other Patient and Public Intervention and Engagement (PPIE) projects. At the start of the project, alongside this I felt a weight of responsibility when meeting Alex Hillman from the research team at my home to discuss the range of questions which could then be put to participants. Quickly I recognised this was not going to be an ordinary research project. It has in fact turned into an extraordinary one, one which has explored creativity through drama – working with the director and actors, and watching the audience reaction; and opera – this time with the composer and librettist and banners – with the artists each taking me and others in the ALWAYs group into areas we had never been before. After a lifetime of avoiding visiting the USA, the IDEAL project gave me the confidence and opportunity to overcome this and when speaking alongside Linda Clare to a packed international auditorium in Chicago, gave me the experience of thanking an audience standing on their feet applauding – the project, not us (sorry Linda!).

I am totally convinced of the importance of evidence-led research and I am often asked to be involved in a new project. One question I ask any team inviting me is around impact and support – both on me and on the project. IDEAL was unique in the amount of time it devoted to this state of nirvana around 'living well with dementia', something which the project explored and the book documents. For me, personally, while life with dementia is getting harder, it is still possible some days for the sun to shine through the cloud and fog and enable me to live as well as possible.

Chapter 12 of this book is probably the most powerfully worded chapter of any book I have read on dementia, and I have read many! I share the research team's vision, and this final chapter clearly outlines the way forward, and could arguably be an appropriate legacy and fitting replacement for the Dementia strategy. The final sentence in the book 'Now is the time to make a change' issues the challenge which, if taken up by those who can make a difference to the lives of people affected by dementia, then the future has hope – again a continual thread in the contributions of those affected by dementia in this amazing book. *Living with Dementia Reconsidered* will sit proudly with its 'siblings' in the *Dementia Reconsidered* book series and is a fitting way to move the work of Tom Kitwood on personhood to greater heights – we have long ago left base camp and the summit is in sight, so let's use this book as our guide to climb upwards.

Acknowledgements

We would like to thank everyone who contributed to the IDEAL research, whether co-investigators, research team members, other university staff, local principal investigators, site researchers, affiliates or advisers, and the many friends and colleagues who have helped and encouraged us along the way. We are grateful to the members of the ALWAYs group and the Project Advisory Group for their support throughout the study. Special thanks go to all the IDEAL participants for sharing their experiences with us.

We are grateful to our funders for making the research possible:

'Improving the experience of Dementia and Enhancing Active Life: living well with dementia. The IDEAL study' was funded jointly by the Economic and Social Research Council (ESRC) and the National Institute for Health and Care Research (NIHR) through grant ES/L001853/2. Investigators: L. Clare, I.R. Jones, C. Victor, J.V. Hindle, R.W. Jones, M. Knapp, M. Kopelman, R. Litherland, A. Martyr, F.E. Matthews, R.G. Morris, S.M. Nelis, J.A. Pickett, C. Quinn, J. Rusted and J. Thom. ESRC is part of UK Research and Innovation (UKRI). IDEAL was registered with the UK Clinical Research Network (UK CRN), registration number 16593, and was approved by Wales Research Ethics Committee 5 (reference 13/WA/0405).

'Improving the experience of Dementia and Enhancing Active Life: a longitudinal perspective on living well with dementia. The IDEAL-2 study' was funded by Alzheimer's Society, grant number 348, AS-PR2-16-001. Investigators: L. Clare, I.R. Jones, C. Victor, C. Ballard, A. Hillman, J.V. Hindle, J. Hughes, R.W. Jones, M. Knapp, R. Litherland, A. Martyr, F.E. Matthews, R.G. Morris, S.M. Nelis, C. Quinn and J. Rusted. IDEAL-2 was registered with UK CRN, registration number 37955, and was approved by Wales Research Ethics Committee 5 (reference 18/WA/0111), Scotland A Research Ethics Committee (reference 18/SS/0037), and the College of Health and Life Sciences Research Ethics Committee at Brunel University London (reference 10598-LR-Mar/2018-12350-2 and 11745-MHR-Jul/2018-13456-2).

'Identifying and mitigating the individual and dyadic impact of COVID19 and life under physical distancing on people with dementia and carers (INCLUDE)' was funded by the Economic and Social Research Council (ESRC) through grant ES/V004964/1. Investigators: L. Clare, C. Victor, F.E. Matthews, C. Quinn, A. Hillman, A. Burns, L. Allan, R. Litherland, A. Martyr, R. Collins, and C. Pentecost. ESRC is part of UK Research and Innovation (UKRI). INCLUDE was approved by Wales Research Ethics Committee 5 as an amendment to IDEAL-2 for England and Wales (18/WS/0111 AM12).

The IDEAL programme was additionally supported by the NIHR Applied Research Collaboration South-West Peninsula.

Recruitment and data collection were conducted from 2014 to 2020 by the following research networks: NIHR Dementias and Neurodegeneration Specialty (DeNDRoN) in England, the Scottish Dementia Clinical Research Network (SDCRN), and Health and Care Research Wales.

The views expressed in this book are those of the authors and not necessarily those of ESRC, UKRI, NIHR, the Department of Health and Social Care, the National Health Service, or Alzheimer's Society.

Abbreviations

ALWAYs	Action on Living Well: Asking You (the IDEAL programme involvement group)
ATM	Automated teller machine (cashpoint)
CFAS-Wales	Cognitive Function and Ageing Study – Wales
CIC	Community interest company
COVID-19	Coronavirus disease 2019 (severe acute respiratory syndrome coronavirus 2)
CRN	Clinical research network
DEEP	Dementia Engagement and Empowerment Project (the UK network of dementia voices)
DFC	Dementia-friendly community
ESRC	Economic and Social Research Council (UK)
G8	Group of Eight (of the world's largest industrial countries)
GP	General practitioner (the UK term for primary care physicians)
GREAT	Goal-oriented cognitive Rehabilitation for Early-stage Alzheimer's and related dementias
HAPI	Health Awareness Profile Interview
IDEAL	Improving the experience of Dementia and Enhancing Active Life
IDEAL-2	The second phase of the IDEAL research programme
MIDAS	Memory Impairment and Dementia Awareness Study
NHS	National Health Service (UK)
NIHR	National Institute of Health and Care Research (UK)
PhD	Doctor of philosophy (doctoral degree)
PPIE	Patient and Public Involvement and Engagement
WHO	World Health Organization

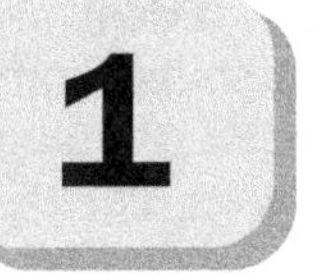

Reconsidering living with dementia: the IDEAL story

Linda Clare

When people get that message, 'I'm sorry to say you have the onset of dementia', the world gets drained out of their head, because it's a death sentence, this is the first thing they think … they decline from that day onwards … and the more they think about it, the more they go into themselves, and the worse they get.

(An IDEAL participant living with dementia)

In this chapter we will:

- explain why we need to rethink living with dementia
- tell the story of the IDEAL research programme
- describe what IDEAL has taught us about living with dementia
- introduce the rest of the book and its calls to action

Why reconsider living with dementia?

Receiving a dementia diagnosis is life-changing. It shapes the course of the rest of that person's life. It has a major impact on close family members and these effects ripple out through the wider network of family and friends. Dementia is the health condition that many people fear the most, and because dementia mainly arises in later life, this fear is compounded by our general reluctance to think about ageing and dying. This can make it difficult for people to think about dementia at all. Yet as individuals and as a society, we need to think about it.

Dementia affects large numbers of mostly older people, who live with the condition often for many years. The number of people worldwide affected by dementia is growing, because we have got better at preventing or treating life-limiting illnesses such as heart disease and because life expectancy is increasing, especially in low- and middle-income countries. Although scientific advances are anticipated, currently there is no cure for any type of dementia, no means of reversing it, and no medical treatment that can stabilise symptoms or prevent progression. There will never be one single cure, or one single approach to treatment or prevention. Dementia is not one condition. The term 'dementia' describes the effects of over 100 different conditions that change how the brain works, affecting an individual's abilities. These conditions have different underlying processes, whether changes in protein metabolism, disruption to the blood supply, or reduced ability to produce vital neurotransmitters. They affect different areas of the brain and involve different patterns of symptoms. Depending on the type of dementia, people might initially experience changes mainly in memory, understanding or use of language, visual perception, movement, personality, or behaviour. Even if advances are made in treating or preventing one type of dementia, and society can afford to implement them, there will still be many people living with the condition for a long time to come.

For many health conditions, cure or improvement in symptoms is the key measure of effective healthcare. With a long-term, progressive, and ultimately terminal neurodegenerative condition such as dementia, good healthcare is important, but it is only one part of the picture. What counts is making sure that people have the best possible experience at every stage and the right support to manage life with the condition. There have been improvements in how we understand and respond to dementia in recent decades. Thanks to the work of Tom Kitwood and others, we are more ready to accept the personhood and citizenship of people with dementia, to acknowledge their human rights, to be inclusive, and to put the person before the disease. With the increasing trend to earlier diagnosis, people with dementia are advocating for themselves and engaging in peer support. Public awareness has grown, and millions of people around the world have become 'Dementia Friends'. Yet there is much more still to do.

People with dementia tell us they need hope to sustain them as they embark on and navigate this journey. Sadly, when they are given their diagnosis, hope is in short supply. Many are sent away with an information leaflet, a helpline number, advice about putting their affairs in order and stopping driving, and perhaps a prescription for a drug that may or may not be helpful, or a referral for a few group sessions. Beyond this they are left to manage alone as symptoms progress and difficulties increase until they eventually reach crisis point. Health services could, should, and sometimes do provide more than this, but the impact of dementia extends way beyond what health services can offer. This is why we need not just to think about dementia, but to rethink the experience of living with dementia.

Dementia is an issue for society, for all of us. How we support vulnerable individuals reflects the kind of society we live in and the values we hold. Providing support for people with dementia acknowledges the contributions they have made throughout their lives to their communities and to society. Even if cost, rather than doing what is right, is the overriding concern, enabling people with dementia and their families to live with the condition, equipping them to manage, and encouraging communities to support them will be more cost-effective than relying on expensive health and social care services. If that is not convincing enough, we should confront the likelihood that many of us reading this will develop dementia in the future if we have not already done so. Before that, we may be called on to support our parents, grandparents, or partners, or perhaps even our children, as they live with dementia. It makes sense for all of us to rethink living with dementia and try to get it right.

The experience of living with dementia

Soon after I started working in the dementia field, I was inspired by Tom Kitwood's book *Dementia Reconsidered* (1997), which explained how a positive and supportive social context not only enhances a person's well-being but also ameliorates the expression of dementia symptoms and vice versa, presenting a strong rationale for sensitive person-centred care. At this time, I was working with experts in brain injury rehabilitation to explore ways of better supporting people with memory difficulties. Rehabilitation is about building on strengths and retained abilities, and compensating for difficulties, in a way that is tailored to the individual and what is important to that person. We had the opportunity to link with a memory clinic and start applying this approach for people recently diagnosed with dementia. We wanted to see whether we could use some of the strategies that work for people whose memory problems arise from brain injury to help people with dementia keep doing the things that are important to them. We found we could, and we have built on that early work to provide evidence that people with dementia and their families can use these strategies to better manage everyday challenges (Clare et al., 2019, 2022).

Kitwood's ideas about how the experience of dementia is shaped by the interplay between the individual and the social context spoke to me especially because they aligned well with the rehabilitative approach. We can distinguish between impairments due to brain pathology, such as memory difficulties in early-stage Alzheimer's, and the impact of these impairments on our ability to carry out activities and participate in society. We may not be able to reverse or cure the impairments, but we can do something about limitations on activity and participation. We can think of this in terms of disability. Disability is not determined just by the nature or extent of impairment; it is influenced by the person's characteristics, relationships, social context, and environment. Social contexts and environments can be disabling and can exclude people from participating. More than this, negative influences can create unnecessary or 'excess' disability – for example, by contributing to the loss of confidence that results in withdrawing from or avoiding activities. This biopsychosocial model of disability (WHO, 2001) is similar to Kitwood's explanation of the way in which a negative social context can undermine well-being while a positive social context can allow the person with dementia to function at the best level possible.

It is often said that if you have met one person with dementia, you have met one person with dementia. Certainly, people respond to the rehabilitation approach in different ways. This made me want to go beyond adapting memory management strategies to understand more about the experience of developing dementia and supporting someone with dementia. I was working with people in the early stages of dementia who could tell me what it felt like. Talking with them and their family members illuminated some of the challenges in adapting to life with the condition, and the many things that influenced their daily lives and sense of well-being. This led to further work, such as the Memory Impairment and Dementia Awareness Study (MIDAS), where we explored how people with early-stage dementia appraised their abilities and difficulties, and the changes they were experiencing (Clare et al., 2011). We talked to over 100 people living with dementia and followed up with as many as possible 12 and 20 months later. We learned a great deal about how people adapt to the condition, but there was a lot still to find out. We needed to paint a complete picture of how personal characteristics, relationships, and social context shape the experience of living with dementia, and how it changes over time as dementia progresses, to help develop policies and practices that make it possible for people to live well with dementia. This was the motivation for developing IDEAL.

Planning the IDEAL programme

IDEAL stands for 'Improving the experience of Dementia and Enhancing Active Life'. The IDEAL research programme ran for 11 years from January 2014 to December 2024. Figure 1.1 shows its structure and timeline. It is unusual for researchers to receive sustained funding enabling them to focus on a topic over a long period, and we did not plan it that way. In 2012, we secured funding for a five-year project, provided jointly by the Economic and Social Research Council (ESRC) and the National Institute for Health and Care Research (NIHR) (Clare et al., 2014). This was part of a competitive call for dementia-related research projects linked to the UK government hosting the Group of Eight (G8) dementia summit in December 2013. As the study got underway and the end of the five-year period came into view, we knew there was a great deal more we could learn

Figure 1.1: Structure and timeline of the IDEAL programme.

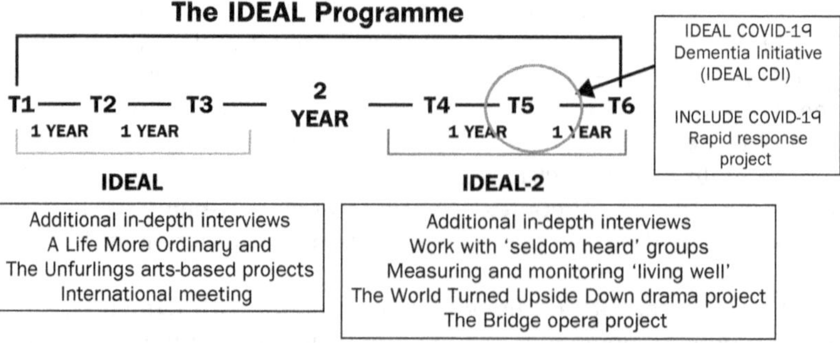

given enough time. When Alzheimer's Society put out a call for large projects including longitudinal studies of quality of life in 2016, we took the opportunity to apply. IDEAL-2 was funded as an Alzheimer's Society Centre of Excellence for five years from 1 January 2018 (Silarova et al., 2018). In the end, this funding was spread over seven years and supplemented by additional grants from NIHR and ESRC which enabled us to investigate the impact of social restrictions during the COVID-19 pandemic between March 2020 and March 2022.

Many people across the UK contributed to IDEAL, as is apparent from Box 1.1. One group I want to mention in particular here is the ALWAYs group. People with dementia and carers were closely involved in developing and shaping the programme from the start. The involvement group we set up in the beginning chose to call themselves the 'Action on Living Well: Asking You' (ALWAYs) group (Litherland et al., 2018). As we journeyed through IDEAL together, the ALWAYs group not only advised, supported, and enthused us but represented IDEAL at conferences, told people about what we found, and got involved in co-producing resources, arts-based activities and outputs to raise public awareness. They were right at the heart of IDEAL and crucial for its success. This book has been developed jointly with them, and two of them created the artwork for the cover.

Box 1.1: Contributors who made IDEAL possible

Leadership team

Co-investigators	19
Affiliates	3

Staff and students

Researcher co-investigators	3
Programme managers	2
Post-doctoral researchers	16
Research assistants	8
Clinical Trials Unit staff	18
Translation and impact specialists	2
Administrators	6
PhD students	4

Contributors across the 34 NHS sites

NHS local Principal Investigators	55
Clinical Research Network (CRN) staff at NHS sites	273

Advisers

ALWAYs group and other advisers	20
Programme advisory groups	21
Liaisons	6

Artists

Lead artists	7
Artists	16

When we started to plan IDEAL, the National Dementia Strategy for England, 'Living Well with Dementia' (Department of Health, 2009), was still fairly new. It set out aspirations to improve attitudes and understanding, promote early diagnosis and intervention, and ensure high-quality care and support to enable people to live well with dementia. We thought that to achieve these aims we needed a better understanding of what it really means to 'live well' with dementia in the community, and of the things that influence the ability to live well with dementia. We set out to build that understanding.

One of our first tasks was to figure out a way of turning the 'living well' concept and the complex set of influences surrounding it into something that could realistically be studied and measured. First, we had to decide what we meant by 'living well' and how to measure it. A report from the Institute of Medicine (2012: 32) described living well with chronic illness as the 'best achievable state of health that encompasses all dimensions of physical, mental and social well-being', and explained that it is shaped by the effect of the illness, the person's physical, social, and cultural surroundings, and the impact on family members, friends, and caregivers. The report emphasised that living well has 'a unique … personal meaning', defined by the person's perceptions of comfort, ability to function, and contentment with life. This description offered a rich framework for exploring living well, emphasising its subjective and personal nature and the influence of relationships, social connections, and the environment. The definition is akin to the World Health Organization (WHO) definition of quality of life as 'an individual's perceptions of their position in life in the context of the culture and values systems in which they live and in relation to their goals, expectations, standards and concerns' (WHOQOL Group, 1994: 28). This views quality of life as a wide-ranging concept, shaped by physical health, psychological state, beliefs and values, and relationships with people and the environment. M. Powell Lawton's influential definition also emphasises the broad nature of the construct, with multiple dimensions of psychological well-being, cognitive and functional ability, and features of the person's environment and living situation all contributing (Lawton, 1994: 138–39). These definitions encompass well-being, the experience of an appropriate balance of positive and negative feelings (Diener et al., 1985; Willroth et al., 2023), and contentment (or satisfaction) with life, an evaluation based on feelings of happiness, meaning, and purpose, a sense of being in control, social participation, and the ability for personal growth (St. John and Montgomery, 2010; Clarke et al., 2020). In IDEAL, we chose to use questionnaires eliciting views about quality of life, well-being, and satisfaction with life to indicate whether people with dementia and carers felt they were living well. Sometimes we combined the three sets of scores statistically to give an overall living well score, and sometimes we used the scores separately.

In the years since the National Dementia Strategy for England set out aspirations about living well in consultation with people affected by dementia, some people with dementia have questioned whether the use of the term 'living well' is helpful. This is because there could be a risk of placing the responsibility for being able to live well solely with the individual, rather than recognising that the challenges and even suffering associated with the condition mean a high level of support is needed to enable people to live well. In IDEAL, we have focused largely on what can help to support people living with the condition, based on the view that the responsibility resides with all of us. I also believe that language matters. There are many negative terms used when talking about dementia, including 'tsunami', 'burden', and 'living death'. You will not find these kinds of terms in this book. 'Living well' is a positive aspiration that fits better with our aims. We will talk more about this in Chapter 3.

Next, we had to decide how to capture the things that could influence living well. We thought that living well would reflect a state of balance where the strengths, resources, and support that people have match or outweigh any challenges they face. Developing dementia, or being a carer for someone with dementia, represents a very significant set of challenges. People approach dementia with different resources, with different strengths, and with access to different degrees of support. They may be better or worse off financially, live in areas with greater or fewer advantages, have better or worse local health services, and so on. These are the social capitals, assets, and resources that people have at their disposal; I will just call them 'resources'. We thought that the interplay between people's resources and the challenges they experience as dementia develops would shape how they adapt and cope, and whether they feel they are living well. We saw adaptation as having two main elements: the way in which people understand and make sense of the condition, and how people evaluate their own situation, capabilities, and needs as the condition develops and progresses.

With these ideas in mind, the questions we posed at the beginning were:

- What does living well mean to people with dementia and carers, and what do they believe helps them to live well or makes it more difficult?
- How do resources, challenges, and adaptation influence capability to live well for both people with dementia and carers?
- How do people with dementia and carers affect each other's ability to live well?
- How does capability to live well change over time, and why?
- What would make it more likely that people with dementia and carers can live well, and how can we encourage people to think differently about dementia?

For IDEAL-2, we had three additional aims. We wanted to understand more about living well for people from minority ethnic groups and explore the experiences of people living with undiagnosed dementia. We will say more about this in Chapter 2. As there was no single measure of living well, we wanted to involve people with dementia in co-producing one. We will say more about this in Chapter 3. Lastly, we wanted to look at ways of including the perspectives of people with more severe dementia. We will say more about this in Chapter 5.

Designing the IDEAL research

We started by looking at what existing research evidence could tell us about influences on living well. We did this by carrying out a systematic review (Martyr et al., 2018). We searched databases containing details of published scientific papers to identify all those containing relevant information. We extracted the statistical information, pooled it, and analysed it all together in a meta-analysis. Few papers focused on well-being or satisfaction with life, so we could only analyse information about quality of life. We included data from 272 journal articles. These articles reported on 198 separate studies, containing information from 37,639 people with dementia. We calculated the statistical links between quality of life scores and 43 possible influences, to see how strongly each of these was connected to a person's quality of life. Somewhat to our surprise, the results did not tell us a great deal.

Most of the influences had small links with perceived quality of life. Only a few stood out. People with strong social connections, good relationships, and better ability to manage everyday activities tended to rate their quality of life more positively. People who had poor mental and physical health, and whose carer had poor well-being, tended to rate their quality of life less favourably. The biggest gap was in understanding what happens to quality of life over time. We wanted to know what would signal that a person's quality of life was likely to decline in the future. This is important because it would suggest what could be changed to help ensure that people with dementia maintain a good quality of life. Unfortunately, the results did not tell us anything useful about this. The review, then, gave us some pointers, but no clear answers. Next, we looked at how best to build on those pointers to get some better answers to our questions.

We wanted to ensure that what we found would influence policy and practice and lead to improvements in the experience of living with dementia. For this to happen, we needed the findings to be both scientifically robust and practically relevant. Given the diverse characteristics and experiences of people affected by dementia, and the number of people affected, we needed to gather information from a large group of people using the same set of questionnaires and applying statistical methods to tease out answers. This meant putting together a survey and sending interviewers to people's homes to go through the questions with them. We were also interested in people's experiences and in the stories that lie behind the numbers. The ALWAYs group members suggested including some open questions alongside the questionnaires, so we asked people to tell us, for example, what 'living well' means to them and what could be changed in their local communities to help them live well. We decided we would go back to a smaller number of the people who completed the questionnaires to have a longer conversation with them and gather their personal stories.

The survey we put together included questions about living well and possible influences on living well. As we thought more about how to understand the answers, we decided to group similar influences on living well together. One important grouping was the personal characteristics of people with dementia. This included things like age, sex, ethnicity, postcode area, housing, and so on. Another was the health and care services people used, and the cost of these services. And another was the quality of the person's relationship with the main family carer (if there was one). Then there were five domains, each covering a set of relevant influences:

- Social situation
- Social capitals, assets, and resources
- Managing everyday life with dementia
- Physical fitness and health
- Psychological characteristics and health

For each domain, we included questionnaires and individual questions asking about various things that might affect living well. For example, under 'physical fitness and health' the topics included how active people were and how much exercise they did, eyesight and hearing, diet and nutrition, and any other illnesses they had. I will say more about the domains later, and each one will be covered in detail in a later chapter.

We intended to let people with dementia speak for themselves, but as we wanted to follow people over time it was possible that some might become less able to answer questions due to the progression of their dementia. We decided to invite each person with dementia who joined the study, if they wished, to nominate a family member or close friend who could join as well. We then asked those individuals to take part in the research and give their views on how they thought the person with dementia was doing. Here we will refer to them as 'carers'. We knew that people with dementia and carers might sometimes see things differently, and we could not just substitute the carer's views if the person with dementia became unable to answer. We thought that by asking carers for their views from the start we would be able to see how and where perspectives differed and take this into account if the time came when the carer was our only source of information. When we later compared the two perspectives, we found that ratings by people with dementia were more positive than carers' ratings, but both sets of ratings had similar links with things that could influence living well, so carers' ratings were still useful (Wu et al., 2020).

We were interested in the carers' own experiences too, and in their capability to live well while caring for someone with dementia. We decided to ask them about living well using similar questions to those asked of the participants with dementia. In most cases, the possible influences on living well and the way we measured them were the same for both people with dementia and carers, but sometimes they differed slightly. For the carers we added a further domain, the experience of being a carer. While in this book we focus mainly on the experiences of people living with dementia, carers play a vital role, and we will talk about what IDEAL has shown us about the experience of being a carer in Chapter 4.

Next, I want to explain how we went about gathering the information to answer our questions.

Developing the IDEAL cohort

At the centre of IDEAL was the cohort study. A cohort study involves recruiting a large group of people and gathering information from them at several points in time. We had to factor in the expectation that some people would withdraw as time went on, owing for example to the dementia getting worse, or to other health problems or changes in circumstances. We estimated that at least one in three would withdraw after two years. Based on our earlier studies and the analyses we planned, we calculated that we needed to recruit 1,500 people with dementia to get robust answers to our questions. We wanted to include people with all types of dementia. We used information from the Dementia UK report (Alzheimer's Society, 2014) about the proportions of people with different dementia diagnoses to confirm that with a sample of 1,500 people we would have enough individuals with each type of dementia remaining in the cohort after two years to allow us to look at them as a group.

We decided to focus on recruiting people in the mild-to-moderate stages of dementia because we wanted to get their views at the start and follow them over time. Adopting an approach that is widely used in dementia research despite its limitations, we considered people scoring 15 or above out of 30 on a screening test called the Mini-Mental State Examination (Folstein et al., 1975) to have mild-to-moderate dementia. We chose to recruit people living in the community rather than those in care homes because we wanted to understand how communities can help to support living well. We also stipulated that participants must be able to give informed consent to take part and should not have another terminal illness, as this would make it difficult to know what was due to dementia and what to the other illness. We wanted to involve a family carer where possible, as I mentioned above, but we thought it was important to include people with dementia who did not have a carer or whose carer did not want to take part. We expected to recruit about 1,050 carers.

What made it possible to set up the cohort study was the support of the NIHR Clinical Research Network (CRN) in England and its equivalents in Scotland and Wales. Network staff embedded in National Health Service (NHS) organisations worked with memory assessment services and other clinics to identify people who could contribute to IDEAL, recruit them, interview them in their own homes (or another place of their choosing), and return the information to the research team. This meant that we could recruit enough people with dementia and carers to achieve our targets.

To thank people for sharing their experiences and giving their time, we offered everyone completing IDEAL interviews at each time point vouchers they could use in a range of shops. To let them know about how the programme was progressing and what we had learned, we kept in touch via twice-yearly newsletters.

Gathering IDEAL data

We partnered initially with 29 NHS organisations throughout England, Scotland, and Wales. CRN staff recruited people to the cohort over a two-year period (mid-2014 to mid-2016) and visited them at home to collect information. To allow enough time to cover everything, the interviews were spread across three visits. We used the data from these Time 1 interviews to look at statistical connections between living well and the things that might influence it when these were all measured at the same time. These are called cross-sectional analyses.

The cohort at Time 1 included 1,537 people with dementia, and the main carer of 1,277 of them. We later added to this, as you will see, so the full cohort consisted of 1,741 people with dementia and 1,452 carers. Among the people with dementia, as Figure 1.2 shows, there were more men than women, although more women than men live with dementia. The proportions of people with each diagnosis were broadly as expected. The cohort consisted mainly of people who identified as white British, which we expected given that ethnic diversity is lowest in older age groups in the UK and people from minority ethnic groups may be less likely to access memory assessment services (Pham et al., 2018). However, they were a diverse group in other ways. They came from a range of social backgrounds and previous occupations. The youngest was aged 43 and the oldest 98. About one in two was dealing with at least one other health condition, and one in five had at least three other health conditions. Use of health services was limited, consisting mainly of outpatient appointments for these other health conditions. Few people made use of social care services and where people did use these, they generally had to pay for them themselves. For the carers, as you can see in Figure 1.3, four out of five were spouses or partners of the person with dementia, and more than one in three were female. The youngest was aged 26 and the oldest 99. These unpaid carers provided most

Figure 1.2: IDEAL cohort participants living with dementia.

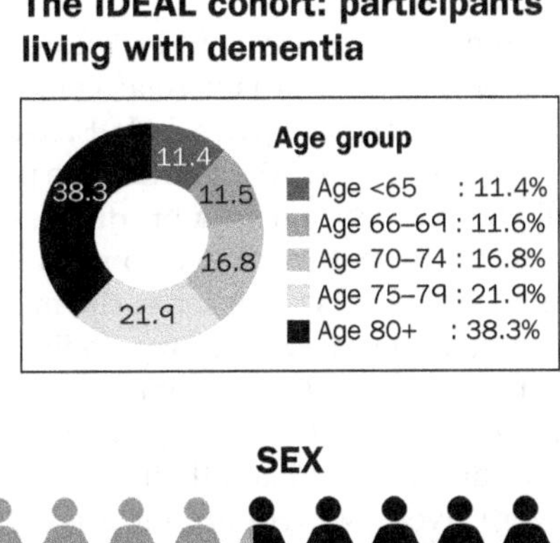

Figure 1.3: Carers of people in the IDEAL cohort who participated in the study.

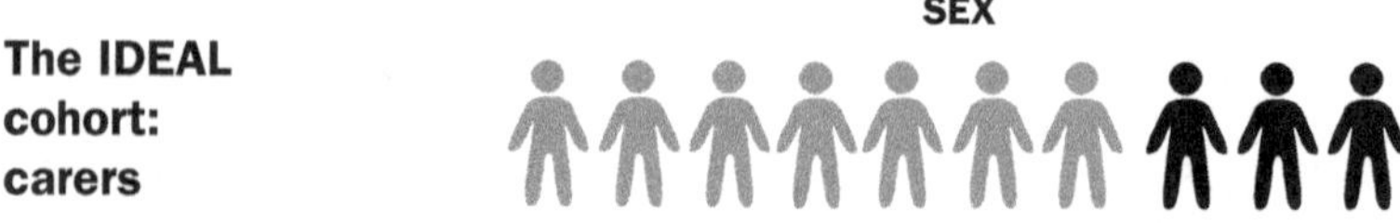

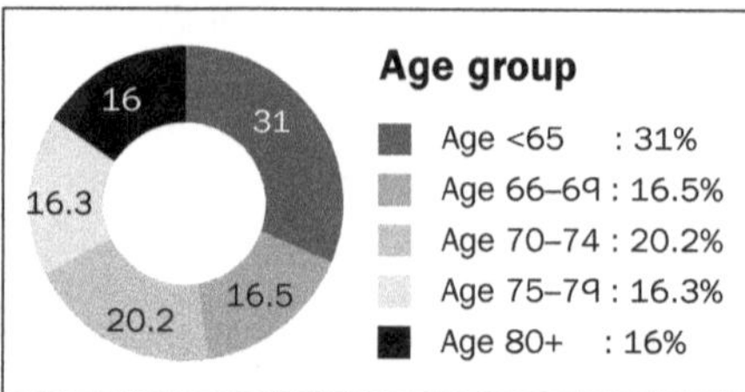

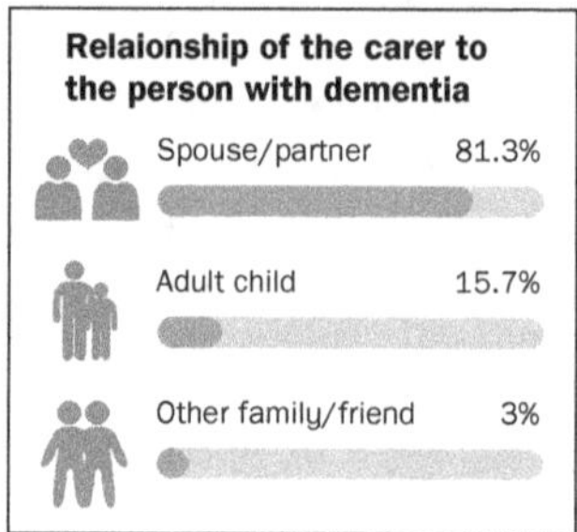

of the support for the participants with dementia. In this chapter, I will focus on the cohort as one group, but in later chapters we will think more about diversity within the cohort and how living well might differ depending on people's situations and characteristics.

Table 1.1 shows how we planned to collect cohort data and what actually happened. With a five-year time frame, we interviewed participants again 12 months and then 24 months after their initial interviews. These interviews were shorter and were spread across two visits. We used the data from all three time points to explore statistically which aspects of people's situation at Time 1 were linked with their capability to live well at Times 2 and 3. These are called longitudinal analyses. With the participants' permission, we could potentially also access health records for both the previous five years and the following five years to see what health services they had received.

Having information from three time points meant we could explore people's experiences over a two-year period. However, this is a relatively short time given that people often live with dementia for many years. In IDEAL-2, we planned to continue interviewing the participants at a further three time points to understand how capability to live well changes as dementia progresses and what influences these changes. In addition, at Time 4 we aimed to recruit 250 new participants, with carers where possible. This was to increase the number of people with Parkinson's disease dementia, dementia with Lewy bodies, and frontotemporal dementia, and people aged either under 65 or 90 and over. These participants were to have their Time 1, 2, and 3 interviews alongside the original participants' Time 4, 5, and 6 rounds so that we could add their information to that already collected. We partnered with five new NHS organisations, and 23 of the original 29 NHS organisations continued to support the study.

We planned IDEAL-2 while Time 2 and Time 3 were in progress, but even so there was an unavoidable two-year gap between Time 3 and Time 4 for each

Table 1.1: IDEAL programme data collection

Time	Dates	Cohort interviews		Conversational interviews	
		People with dementia	**Carers**	**People with dementia**	**Carers**
Time 1	*Planned:* Mid-2014 to mid-2016 + Mid-2018 to mid-2020 *Actual:* Mid-2014 to mid-2016 + Mid-2018 to Feb 2020	1537 + 204 = 1741	1277 + 175 = 1452	5 ALWAYs group members	4 ALWAYs group members
Time 2	*Planned:* Mid-2015 to mid-2017 + Mid-2019 to mid-2021 *Actual:* Mid-2015 to mid-2017 + Mid-2019 to Feb 2020	1183 + 43 = 1226	998 + 41 = 1039	20 Cohort participants	20 Cohort participants
Time 3	*Planned:* Mid-2016 to mid-2018 + Mid-2020 to mid-2022 *Actual:* Mid-2016 to mid-2018 + April 2022 to Dec 2022	851 + 40 = 891	759 + 69 = 828	17 Cohort participants	14 Cohort participants
Time 4	*Planned:* Mid-2018 to mid-2020 *Actual:* Mid-2018 to Feb 2020	253	237		
Time 5	*Planned:* Mid-2019 to mid-2021 *Actual:* Mid-2019 to Feb 2020	31	31		
COVID-19	Sep 2021 to April 2022 May to July 2020 Nov to Dec 2020 Jan to April 2021 Dec 2021 to Jan 2022	173	242	11 11 7 9	11 10 7 10
Time 6	*Planned:* Mid-2020 to mid-2022 *Actual:* April 2022 to Dec 2022	96	170	5 Cohort participants	4 Cohort participants

person. Times 4 to 6 were scheduled for mid-2018 to mid-2022. This turned out not to be the best timing. The arrival of the COVID-19 pandemic in early 2020 put an end to visiting participants at home, disrupting Times 4 and 5. We rapidly changed our approach and set up a round of interviews conducted by the research team via telephone or video call. We knew that some people might find this challenging, but it was the only way we could keep in touch with cohort participants. The ALWAYs group helped us work out how to do the interviews in a way that people would find manageable. These interviews, carried out between September 2020 and April 2021, focused mainly on the impact of the pandemic but also covered some of the missing Time 5 information. With the pandemic ongoing, we opted to do the Time 6 interviews in the same way from May to December 2021.

We asked a small number of cohort participants to meet a researcher for a conversation about their experiences. Members of the ALWAYs group volunteered to help us test the approach. For these conversational interviews, we chose to invite people with dementia whose scores for living well changed between Time 1 and Time 2, together with their carers, so that we could explore what might lie behind these changes. We met as many as possible again a year later. At Time 6, we went back to see as many as possible a third time, four years after the previous meeting. During the COVID-19 period, we did three extra rounds of telephone interviews with people with dementia and their carers to find out about their experiences during the pandemic and how the social restrictions had affected them.

Living with dementia in the IDEAL cohort

At their first meeting, the Project Advisory Group gave us some valuable advice. They thought we should start by looking at the overall influences on living well for people with dementia and try to paint a full picture before going into detail about specific topics. We did this with the Time 1 data (Clare et al., 2019), using information about five domains:

- Social situation
- Social capitals, assets, and resources
- Managing everyday life with dementia
- Physical fitness and health
- Psychological characteristics and health

For each domain, we measured several topics using questionnaires and individual questions; I will call these 'measures'. We first looked at which measures were statistically linked to living well scores; that is, whether better or worse scores on a measure were reliably coupled with better or worse scores for living well. Then, for each domain, we took the measures whose scores were linked with living well, statistically derived a single combined score, and estimated how strongly that score was related to the living well score. All the domains were meaningfully related to living well. In Figure 1.4, the grey bars show how strong these connections were. A more positive social situation, greater social resources, better physical health, and better psychological health were all linked to higher living well scores and vice versa. This told us that it was right to think broadly about influences on capability to live well, but it was not the end of the story.

The final step in building the overall picture was to see what happened when we took all five domains together and analysed how they related to living well, in effect allowing them to compete against each other. The black bars in Figure 1.4 show that when we did this, the psychological domain dominated as the most closely related to living well. This confirms that people's subjective experience is important, but it does not mean that other domains are irrelevant. A better way of looking at this is to understand that social situation, social resources, physical health, and managing the everyday challenges of dementia all influence how people feel about themselves, their emotions, and their mental health, which in turn is strongly linked to whether they see themselves as living well. Therefore, to promote living well, it is not enough to focus just on dementia symptoms; we need to think about all these aspects of people's lives.

We looked at what people with dementia said when asked 'What does living well mean to you?', to see how it fitted with this overall picture (Quinn et al., 2022). What they told us mapped onto the social, physical, psychological, and managing life with dementia domains. We will say more about this in Chapter 3. It confirmed that we should be thinking about all these aspects of people's lives. Together, this information gave us the basis of our 'Living with Dementia Map' for people with dementia, a visual representation of the influences on living well.

The next step was to find out how things changed over time and whether anything in people's scores at Time 1 could signal the likelihood that their capability to live well would change. We first used the data from Times 1, 2, and 3, and to make the analyses more manageable we used quality of life as the

Figure 1.4: Relationship of life domains to living well.

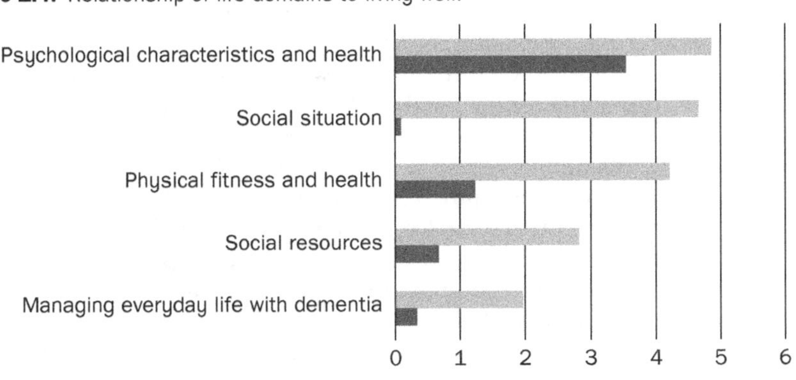

indicator of living well (Clare et al., 2022), although the results for well-being and satisfaction with life were similar. There was little change in quality of life over the two-year period; scores stayed the same for almost nine out of ten people with dementia (88.6 per cent). One reason could be that the people who continued in the study were doing better than those who withdrew. We found that those who withdrew were slightly older and had slightly more cognitive difficulties than those who continued, and scored slightly lower for living well, but generally the differences were small, so this was not enough to explain why we found such a stable pattern.

The group of people with stable scores included a majority (74.9 per cent) with scores suggesting reasonably good quality of life and a smaller group (13.7 per cent) with markedly lower scores. People with lower quality of life scores had poorer Time 1 scores for social situation, physical health, ability to manage everyday activities, and psychological health than those with higher scores. These low scores were already well established when we first talked to people and stayed the same two years later. For people in this group, efforts to improve capability to live well by focusing on these areas where people were doing poorly need to start from the time of diagnosis.

Of the people whose quality of life scores changed, a small proportion whose initial scores suggested reasonable quality of life (7.6 per cent) rated their quality of life lower over time. They were lonelier and more depressed, had lower self-esteem, and felt less optimistic at Time 1 than those whose scores stayed the same. This suggests what might alert us to the risk of decline in living well and what could be done to ensure that people maintain their capability to live well.

An even smaller proportion of participants with initially low quality of life scores (3.8 per cent) improved over time. These people did slightly less well on memory tests at Time 1 than those whose scores remained low but were not different in other ways. This did not give us any pointers about what leads to improvement in scores.

We extended the analyses with information from Times 4, 5, and 6. We looked at quality of life scores over time with date of diagnosis as the starting point. In general, self-ratings of quality of life by people with dementia did not change much, although carers' ratings of the person's quality of life declined. There were some people with dementia, however, whose scores did decline. When people got more depressed or rated their health as poorer, this tended to be followed by a drop in quality of life. We saw this drop in quality of life more often in people aged under 80 than in those aged 80 and over (Clare et al., 2023).

This added the remaining details to our Living with Dementia Map (IDEAL Programme, n.d.), shown in Figure 1.5. It emphasizes again that how people feel about themselves is crucial for living well and is shaped by many aspects of their lives. Increased depression and other signs of poor psychological well-being, and a feeling of being in worse health, can alert us that a drop in capability to live well is likely. While I have focused here on people with dementia, we explored carers' experiences in a similar way, and we will say more about this in Chapter 4.

Figure 1.5: Living with Dementia Map for people with dementia.

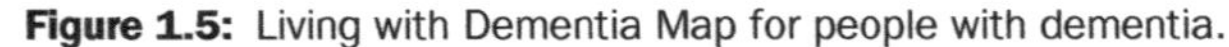

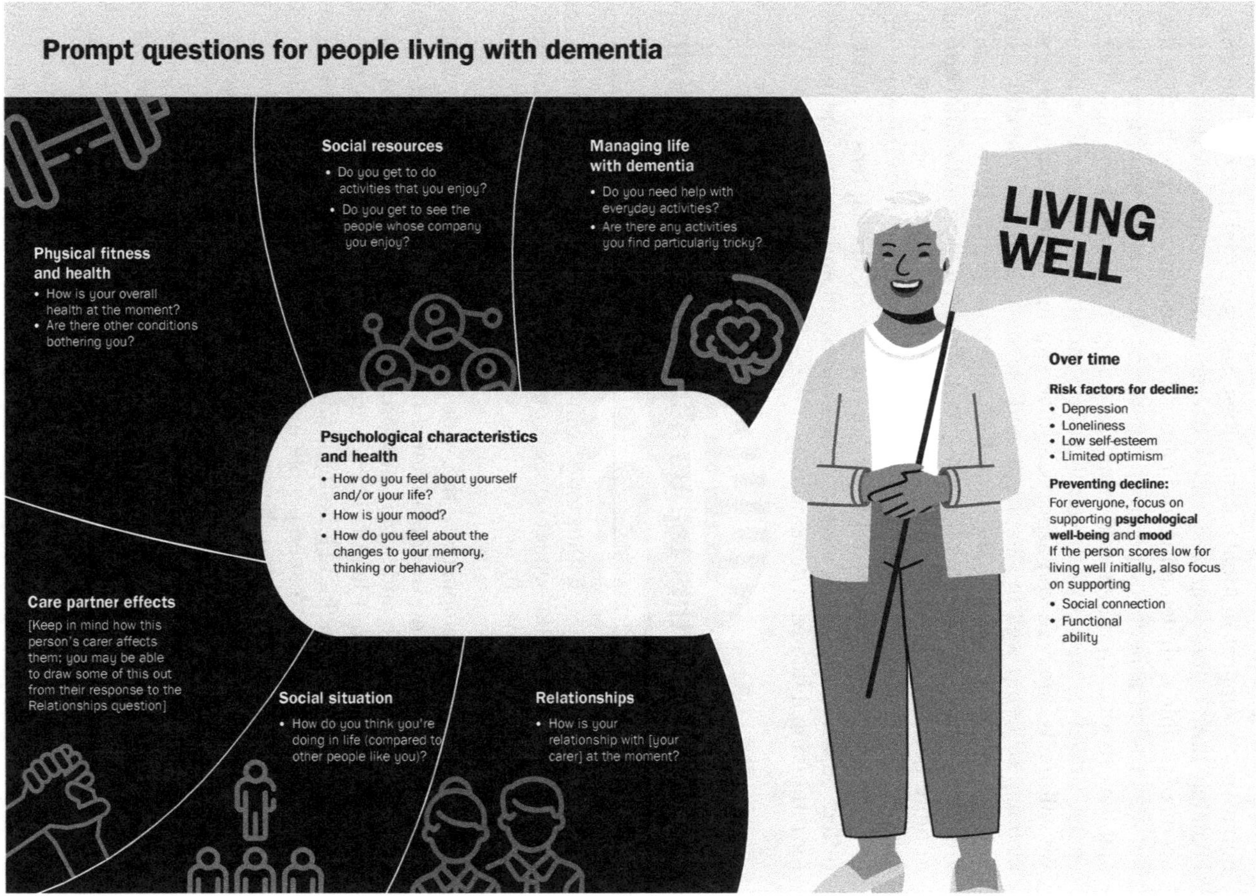

What we have learned gives us an overall picture of what makes it easier or harder to live well with dementia. This is something that policy-makers can use when thinking about what health and social care services are needed and what initiatives to support in local communities. Service providers can use it when planning how to develop services and community resources that meet the needs of people with dementia and carers. Practitioners can use it when thinking about what aspects of people's experience they might want to ask about and how to identify things that could be changed to improve people's experiences. However, within this overall picture there is a great deal of diversity. We will focus on some key aspects of diversity in Chapter 2, on the personal meaning of living well in Chapter 3, and on the vital role of unpaid, usually family carers in Chapter 4. The overall picture tells us about the wide range of life domains that are relevant for living well. We will look at individual domains in more detail in Chapters 5 to 9 and examine the role that services play in Chapter 10. Throughout, we will focus on what could improve the experience of living with dementia and draw out calls for action. In Chapters 11 and 12, we reflect on what IDEAL has meant to those involved and present our manifesto for rethinking living with dementia.

So what does this tell us about reconsidering living with dementia?

I started by saying that, with a long-term progressive neurodegenerative condition such as dementia, what counts is making sure people can live as well as possible at every stage. To achieve this, we need to reconsider what it means to live with dementia.

IDEAL findings demonstrate the wide range of things that make a difference to living well and the importance of a socially oriented understanding alongside good health and social care provision. The centrality of psychological characteristics and health is encouraging because how people feel can potentially change. Tackling loneliness and depression, and fostering hope and self-efficacy, can help to keep people living well. However, this should not be misunderstood as suggesting the problem lies in the individual and needs to be 'fixed' through, for example, medication for depression. How people feel is shaped by what they have experienced and are experiencing. There may be things we cannot change, but some aspects linked with poorer capability to live well could potentially be changed, especially by tackling social disadvantage and improving environments and services, supporting social connections, and enabling people to better manage everyday life with dementia. For example, tacking social isolation might require various approaches, including improving transport links and accessibility of venues, developing dementia supportive activities in local areas, equipping people with practical strategies to enable them to engage, and reaching out and offering support to overcome lack of confidence.

We need the right policies, structures, services, and support in place to enable people to live well. The IDEAL Living with Dementia Map presents the voice and experience of people with dementia and carers to policy-makers, commissioners of services, service providers, and practitioners in a way that is intended to help them rethink living with dementia. This is the basis for the call to action set out in this book.

Key points

Key points for people with dementia and carers

- Living with dementia or caring for someone living with dementia is challenging and people need support to live well with the condition.
- There is hope that you can live well with dementia.
- There are resources and support available, and you will read about some of them in this book.

Key points for practitioners and providers

- Many aspects of people's lives influence capability to live well with dementia.
- Focus on promoting psychological, physical, and social health.
- Address what is important to each person and equip them to manage the challenges of living with or supporting someone with dementia.

Key points for policy-makers

- Many aspects of people's lives influence capability to live well with dementia.
- Dementia is not just a medical issue – a socially oriented, inclusive approach should be a cornerstone of policy development.
- Practical support for unpaid carers is crucial.

References

Alzheimer's Society (2014) *Dementia UK: Update,* 2nd edition. London: Alzheimer's Society. Available at: https://www.alzheimers.org.uk/sites/default/files/migrate/downloads/dementia_uk_update.pdf (accessed 10 September 2024).

Clare, L., Whitaker, C.J., Nelis, S.M., et al. (2011) Multi-dimensional assessment of awareness in early-stage dementia: a cluster analytic approach, *Dementia and Geriatric Cognitive Disorders,* 31(5): 317–27.

Clare, L., Nelis, S.M, Quinn, C., et al. (2014) Improving the experience of dementia and enhancing active life – living well with dementia: study protocol for the IDEAL study, *Health and Quality of Life Outcomes,* 12:164. Available at: https://doi.org/10.1186/s12955-014-0164-6.

Clare, L., Wu, Y.-T., Jones, I.R., et al. (2019) A comprehensive model of factors associated with subjective perceptions of 'living well' with dementia: findings from the IDEAL study, *Alzheimer Disease and Associated Disorders*, 33(1): 36–41.

Clare, L., Gamble, L.D., Martyr, A., et al. (2022) Longitudinal trajectories of quality of life among people with mild-to-moderate dementia: a latent growth model approach with IDEAL cohort study data, *Journals of Gerontology B: Psychological Sciences and Social Sciences*, 77(6): 1037–50.

Clare, L., Gamble, L.D., Martyr, A., et al. (2023) Longitudinal factors associated with living well in people with mild-to-moderate dementia, *Innovation in Aging*, 7(suppl. 1): 433–34.

Clarke, C., Woods, B., Moniz-Cook, E., et al. (2020) Measuring the well-being of people with dementia: a conceptual scoping review, *Health and Quality of Life Outcomes*, 18(1): 249. Available at: https://doi.org/10.1186/s12955-020-01440-x.

Department of Health (2009) *Living well with dementia: A national dementia strategy*. London: Department of Health. Available at: https://www.gov.uk/government/publications/living-well-with-dementia-a-national-dementia-strategy (accessed 10 September 2024).

Diener, E., Emmons, R.A., Larsen, R.J., et al. (1985) The satisfaction with life scale, *Journal of Personality Assessment*, 49(1): 71–75.

Folstein, M.F., Folstein, S.E. and McHugh, P.R. (1975) 'Mini-mental state': a practical method for grading the cognitive state of patients for the clinician, *Journal of Psychiatric Research*, 12(3): 189–98.

IDEAL Programme (n.d.) *Living with Dementia Maps*. Available at: https://www.ideal-project.org.uk/projects/maps/ (accessed 14 September 2024).

Institute of Medicine (2012) *Living well with chronic illness: A call for public health action*. Washington, DC: National Academies Press. Available at: https://nap.nationalacademies.org/catalog/13272/living-well-with-chronic-illness-a-call-for-public-health (accessed 10 September 2024).

Kitwood, T. (1997) *Dementia Reconsidered: The Person Comes First*. Buckingham: Open University Press.

Lawton, M.P. (1994) Quality of life in Alzheimer disease, *Alzheimer Disease and Associated Disorders*, 8(suppl. 3): 138–50.

Litherland, R., Burton, J., Cheeseman, M., et al. (2018) Reflections on PPI from the 'Action on Living Well: Asking You' advisory network of people with dementia and carers as part of the IDEAL study, *Dementia*, 17(8): 1035–44.

Martyr, A., Nelis, S.M., Quinn, C., et al. (2018) Living well with dementia: a systematic review and correlational meta-analysis of factors associated with quality of life, well-being and life satisfaction in people with dementia, *Psychological Medicine*, 48(13): 2130–39.

Pham, T.M., Petersen, I., Walters, K., et al. (2018) Trends in dementia diagnosis rates in UK ethnic groups: analysis of UK primary care data, *Clinical Epidemiology*, 10: 949–60.

Quinn, C., Pickett, J.A., Litherland, R., et al. (2022) Living well with dementia: what is possible and how to promote it, *International Journal of Geriatric Psychiatry*, 37(1): e5627. Available at: https://doi.org/10.1002/gps.5627.

Silarova, B., Nelis, S.M., Ashworth, R.M., et al. (2018) Protocol for the IDEAL-2 longitudinal study: following the experiences of people with dementia and their primary carers to understand what contributes to living well with dementia and enhances active life, *BMC Public Health*, 18(1): 1214. Available at: https://.doi.org/10.1186/s12889-018-6129-7.

St. John, P.D. and Montgomery, P.R. (2010) Cognitive impairment and life satisfaction in older adults, *International Journal of Geriatric Psychiatry*, 25(8): 814–21.

WHOQOL Group (1994) Development of the WHOQOL: rationale and current status, *International Journal of Mental Health*, 23(3): 24–56.

Willroth, E.C., Pfund, G.N., McGhee, C., et al. (2023) Well-being as a protective factor against cognitive decline and dementia: a review of the literature and directions for future research, *Journals of Gerontology B: Psychological Sciences and Social Sciences*, 78(5): 765–76.

World Health Organization (WHO) (2001) *International Classification of Impairments, Disabilities and Handicaps*. Geneva: WHO. Available at: https://www.who.int/standards/classifications/international-classification-of-functioning-disability-and-health (accessed 10 August 2024).

Wu, Y.-T., Nelis, S.M., Quinn, C., et al. (2020) Factors associated with self- and informant ratings of quality of life, well-being and life satisfaction in people with mild-to-moderate dementia: results from the Improving the experience of Dementia and Enhancing Active Life programme, *Age and Ageing*, 49(3): 446–52.

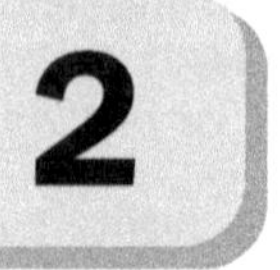

Dementia has many meanings: identity and diversity

Linda Clare

In this chapter we will:

- explore differences in the experience of living with dementia
- find out how living well varies by type and severity of dementia
- examine who is disadvantaged in access to services and capability to live well
- consider whether different ways of understanding dementia affect living well

Diversity and inclusion

We are all different. We start life with different characteristics and traits, and these are shaped by experience over our lifetime. We have different values, beliefs, capabilities, interests, likes, and dislikes. This is as true of people with dementia as for any other group. Understanding and accepting this diversity and becoming more inclusive is central to rethinking the experience of living with dementia.

Often in research we try to iron out differences statistically to get a clear picture that applies across the board. In many IDEAL analyses looking at what influences living well, we ironed out, or 'controlled for', differences due to age or sex. That way we can be more confident that the differences that remain reflect the influences we are exploring. This is valuable when we want to understand the big picture but needs to be balanced with appreciation of differences and their impact.

Living well with dementia is about much more than getting a diagnosis and managing symptoms. Our 'Living with Dementia Map', introduced in Chapter 1, shows that social situation, social resources, psychological well-being, and physical health are all important. The way in which these influences play out in our daily lives will vary, and what is most relevant for living well will differ between individuals and groups. In IDEAL, we have been able to draw out some of these individual differences. The main aim of this chapter, though, is to look at the differences we can see when we group together people with dementia who share a similar characteristic or set of characteristics and compare them to others who do not share the same characteristics. This allows policy and practice to consider diversity and be more inclusive. This is central to rethinking the experience of living with dementia.

Here, I will think about diversity from three perspectives: differences due to dementia, differences arising from who we are, and differences linked to how we understand the condition.

Differences due to dementia

Different dementias are different.

(Keith, ALWAYs group member)

We often talk about 'dementia' as if it is one thing, but this is misleading. 'Dementia' describes the effects of over 100 different conditions. Each develops and progresses gradually, and rates of change vary both across conditions and among individuals with each condition. People's experiences and needs for support change as the condition progresses, whether slowly over several years or more rapidly. The experience of living with dementia is shaped among other things by the type, nature, and severity of the person's condition.

Researchers sometimes opt to study people with a specific type of dementia, typically Alzheimer's disease. We wanted to explore the experiences of people with all types of dementia. In the IDEAL cohort, just over half of the people with dementia had a diagnosis of Alzheimer's disease, one in ten had vascular dementia, and one in five had mixed Alzheimer's and vascular dementia. Around 3 in 100 had either frontotemporal dementia, Parkinson's disease dementia, Lewy body dementia, or another diagnosis. When we compared scores on measures of living well (Wu et al., 2018), people with Alzheimer's disease or frontotemporal dementia gave the most positive ratings, people with vascular or mixed dementia provided slightly lower ratings, while people with Parkinson's disease dementia and Lewy body dementia gave the lowest ratings of all. Differences between the groups on measures of living well remained the same over time (Martyr et al., 2024).

These differences in living well ratings were reflected in differences in the health and social care services people received, and in the cost of these services. Initially, costs were three times higher for people with Parkinson's disease dementia, and half as much again for people with Lewy body dementia, when compared to people with Alzheimer's disease (Henderson et al., 2019). Over time, costs increased most steeply for people with Lewy body or frontotemporal dementia (Henderson et al., 2022). There could be several reasons for this. People with Parkinson's disease dementia will probably have been in contact with specialist Parkinson's services before developing dementia, have a named Parkinson's specialist nurse, and be receiving medical treatment for movement-related symptoms. People with Lewy body dementia may also access specialised treatment for the challenging symptoms and more rapid changes in mental or 'cognitive' ability associated with this type of dementia. Similarly, the symptoms experienced by people with frontotemporal dementia could lead to more contact with services. People with Parkinson's disease dementia were more likely than those with Alzheimer's to say they received support from services (van Horik et al., 2022). They were also more likely to move into a care home (Sabatini et al., 2024).

Next, I want to turn to differences due to severity of dementia. IDEAL evidence is mostly relevant to people living with mild-to-moderate dementia. Three-quarters of those remaining in the cohort by Time 4 were still in the mild-to-moderate stage. Living well is equally important for people whose dementia has progressed further, and we wanted to explore this too. We started with a focus on communication, which we will talk about in Chapter 5, because we needed to think about the best ways of gathering the views of people whose dementia had progressed further. Unfortunately, we could not talk to people with more severe dementia as part of IDEAL due to the COVID-19 pandemic. Instead, we decided to draw together what research has already told us about living well as dementia becomes more severe.

Studies conducted in residential long-term care settings emphasise that social contact is central to quality of life. People with severe dementia initiate and respond to contact and can identify things they enjoy (Mayhew et al., 2001) but often lack meaningful social contact and talk of missing their family and home, and of feeling lonely, or even hopeless and despairing (Clare et al., 2008; Cahill and Diaz-Ponce, 2011). Social contact that promotes personhood is vital. Alongside this, while people with mild-to-moderate dementia value structured activities or outings, for people with more severe dementia small pleasures such as a good cup of tea or a nice chat seem more important for quality of life (Cahill and Diaz-Ponce, 2011).

In rethinking the experience of living with dementia, we need to remember that it differs markedly depending on the type and severity of the condition. It is time to acknowledge this diversity and to ensure that we support people with dementia by gaining more specialised understanding of the types of dementia and of the needs people have at each stage of progression. But these are not the only dimensions of difference that we need to keep in mind.

Differences due to who we are

> *Dementia doesn't just alter by type. It's altered by the environment.*
> (Jane, ALWAYs group member)

Just as it is misleading to talk about dementia as if it is one condition, it is equally misleading to talk about 'people with dementia' as if everyone with dementia is the same. The experience of living with the condition and the support people get differs depending on who they are and where they live.

At Time 1, we asked IDEAL participants and their carers about the support that people with dementia received after a dementia diagnosis. The WHO global action plan encourages all countries to find ways to meet the care and support needs of people with dementia and carers (WHO, 2017). In England, guidelines current at the time of writing (NICE, 2018) say that people with dementia should receive accessible information about their condition, have a named health or social care professional responsible for co-ordinating their care, receive evidence-based treatments to address clinical needs, and have support to engage in activities that reflect their personal preferences and needs.

In IDEAL, just under half of the participants with dementia said they had received information about their condition. Three-quarters of the carers said the person with dementia had been given information. Fewer than one in three people with dementia, and just over one in three carers, thought there was a named professional in place for the person with dementia. Some answers suggested that a named professional was in contact due to another health condition. Similarly, fewer than one in three people with dementia, and one in three carers, said the person with dementia had received any treatment other than medication. The people most likely to respond positively to these questions were relatively young and well-educated males.

This shows that support following diagnosis was low across the board. This could mean that services were not available, or that available services were not used because they were difficult to access or seen as unhelpful. We found no evidence that older women are less likely to receive a diagnosis, but it seems they are less likely to receive support (van Horik et al., 2022). Health and social care costs for women with dementia were lower than those for men with dementia (Henderson et al., 2019), although this difference reduced over time (Henderson et al., 2022).

Older women with dementia are more likely than others to live alone (Clare et al., 2020). In the IDEAL cohort, just under 1 in 20 people with dementia were living alone, and this included a relatively high proportion of women aged over 80. People living alone had fewer difficulties with memory and with everyday activities, were more independent than those living with others, and were more likely to use domestic help and equipment such as falls prevention and mobility aids. However, they were more depressed and lonelier than those living with others, had poorer health, and scored poorer on measures of living well. Over time, their quality of life declined relative to those living with others, and they were more likely to move into a care home (Clare et al., 2024).

This suggests that discrimination based on ageist and sexist attitudes could be contributing to inequalities in receiving services. Ethnicity is another dimension that could affect the experience of living with dementia. While the big picture in the living well map is probably relevant across many contexts, both the relative emphasis on individual domains and what is most important within those domains could vary for people of different ethnicities. The

IDEAL cohort were mostly white British. The proportion of older people from minority ethnic groups is still relatively small in the UK, but this will change. It is important to think about living well for people from minority ethnic groups, both to improve people's experience now and to plan inclusive provision in the future.

We looked at the experiences of 20 people in the cohort who were of Indian, Pakistani, Bangladeshi, black African or Caribbean, or mixed ethnicity (Victor et al., 2024a). We matched the information from each of them with information from three white British cohort members with similar characteristics, allowing us to compare two groups that were similar apart from their ethnicity. The people with dementia from minority ethnic groups had poorer quality of life than their white counterparts and felt lonelier. Although our participants of black, Asian, or mixed heritage were a small and diverse group, this does suggest that when it comes to living with dementia, as in many other aspects of life, people from minority ethnic groups are at a disadvantage.

To understand this better, we talked with people with dementia, carers, and community leaders from these ethnic groups (Victor et al., 2024b). First-generation migrants had a sense of not belonging and not being full members of society; many had expected to return home but ended up staying in the country where they had built their lives and where their children had settled. Experiences of racism and discrimination had shaped the course of their lives and presented barriers to achievement. These barriers and the resulting lack of trust also extended to accessing services, where they found themselves '*ten steps behind*'. Services for people with dementia were difficult to access (especially for those who speak no or limited English), were sometimes of poor quality, and lacked sensitivity to cultural needs. The same was true of care settings, which failed to provide familiar food or culturally sensitive personal care. Other reasons for not accessing services, especially among the Asian community, were the stigma attached to symptoms of dementia and a belief that changes in memory were a normal feature of ageing. The Hamari Yaadin (Our Memories) banner made by the Touchstones group in Leeds, in northern England as part of our Unfurlings arts-based project described in detail in Chapter 3, and shown in Figure 2.1, asks: 'When we talk, will you listen?'

This combination of low expectations of services and beliefs about dementia-related changes being a normal part of getting older also emerged when we talked to another group not accessing dementia services – people living with undiagnosed dementia. In England, in 2023, it was estimated that only about two-thirds of people experiencing dementia had received a diagnosis. Diagnosis is seen as providing a gateway to services and support, although as we have already noted post-diagnostic support is limited. There are various reasons why people might not have a diagnosis – for example, they might not consult a doctor at all, or if they do, their difficulties might be put down to something else, or considered too mild to warrant a referral for assessment. In the second stage of IDEAL, as part of our focus on including diverse groups, we wanted to find out more about people living with undiagnosed dementia.

Figure 2.1: Hamari Yaadin banner 'When we talk, will you listen?'

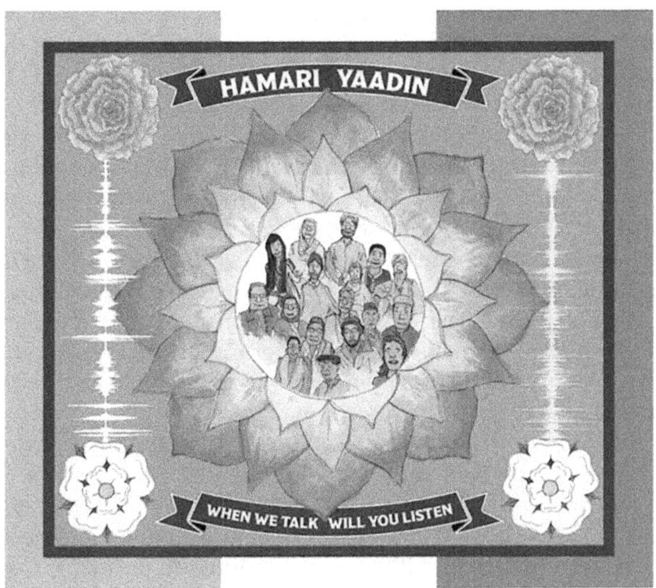

The IDEAL team was involved with another British cohort where we could expect to find people living with undiagnosed dementia, the Cognitive Function and Ageing Study Wales (CFAS-Wales). The CFAS-Wales cohort was a representative sample of the population aged 65+ in two areas of Wales. We could identify people whose scores showed that they had dementia and check their general practitioner (GP) records to see whether they had a diagnosis of dementia. There were 19 people whose scores indicated they had dementia and who also had a diagnosis, and 105 people whose scores indicated they had dementia but who did not have a diagnosis.

We looked for obvious differences between the people living with undiagnosed dementia and those with a diagnosis (Gamble et al., 2022). People in the undiagnosed group were better educated and had better scores on cognitive tests. This makes sense, because they might still be managing well day-to-day; if they did seek help, they might do reasonably well on standard screening tests and difficulties might only show up on more detailed testing, which is not always available. People in the undiagnosed group were more likely to be experiencing depression. Again, this makes sense because depression is common in the early stages of dementia and the effects of depression can be similar to dementia-related changes, so treating depression first could be a reasonable strategy. People in the undiagnosed group were more likely to live in less well-off areas. Services in these areas could be less well-resourced and less trusted, meaning that people either cannot access help or do not seek help because they have low expectations.

As part of a CFAS-Wales follow-up, without referring to 'dementia', we talked to six of the individuals with undiagnosed dementia and their family carers (Henley et al., 2021). We also talked to four family carers of three people with undiagnosed dementia who were now living in care homes. Three main insights emerged. First, people focused on the impact of physical health problems, mobility difficulties, and sensory impairments. They saw memory and other cognitive difficulties as a normal aspect of getting older, and something to which they could adapt. Second, people relied on informal help and support and took pride in managing without the need for outside help or professional involvement. Third, people were reluctant to visit the doctor. They found it difficult to get appointments, disliked having to see a different doctor at each visit, and expected little in the way of support from under-resourced services. Negative perceptions of services and beliefs about dementia combined to shape how people in this undiagnosed group responded to developing dementia symptoms.

What this exploration of diversity tells us is that aspects of who we are – those I have focused on here and undoubtedly also many others – affect the experience of living with dementia just as they affect our lives in general. Further IDEAL analyses showed that age, education, income, home ownership, and living situation (alone or with others) combine to influence quality of life for people with dementia. Those who fared best were older homeowners with educational qualifications and higher incomes who lived with others. People who were younger, had no educational qualifications, lived alone, and were not homeowners fared least well. This highlights the need for targeted efforts to reduce inequalities. In rethinking living with dementia, we can and should work to change the structures and attitudes that underlie unequal access to resources. We can potentially improve the quality of services and equip them to offer personalised and culturally sensitive support. Alongside this, there is a need to build or rebuild trust and acknowledge the impact of accumulated negative experiences on attitudes and expectations. The other important point that emerges is the need for a shared understanding of dementia that makes it as easy as possible for people to access support while avoiding stigma and maintaining well-being.

Differences due to how we understand dementia

What a person thinks about dementia = what you're actually told + what you've experienced in your life + your own knowledge + your personality.
(Jane, ALWAYs group member)

How people understand a health condition influences how they cope with it. How people cope with a health condition makes a difference to how well they do, separate from the effects of the condition itself. We all have beliefs about various health conditions, developed through our experience, through what we observe, and through what we learn from TV, movies, books, newspapers, and social media. When we notice symptoms and feel our own health is threatened, those beliefs are the starting point for understanding what is happening and deciding what to do about it.

As we develop a health condition, our beliefs evolve through our experiences and the knowledge and information we gather into a mental picture, or representation, of the condition. This summarises our understanding of the condition, and includes the nature, cause, and course of the illness, its practical and emotional consequences, and what can be done to control it. This 'illness representation' shapes how we feel about the condition and what we do in response to it (Hagger and Orbell, 2022). Faced with the same health condition, people with different representations will react and cope in different ways, whether helpful or unhelpful. Those who usually cope by focusing on how they feel might dwell on the frustration that it causes or find it so threatening that they avoid thinking about it altogether, making it difficult to manage the effects of the condition or to seek help. People who typically cope by tackling and trying to solve problems might try to improve things by seeking advice, adopting a healthier lifestyle, or devising strategies to compensate for difficulties. People usually feel better if they think there are things they can do to try to deal with a problem, and this helps with managing the condition.

We thought this could be relevant for understanding the experience of people living with dementia. Dementia is one of the health conditions people are most afraid of developing. Across cultures it is linked with stigma, and even associated with madness or witchcraft. Someone developing dementia might experience this as a threat to their identity. One survey conducted by Alzheimer's Society in the UK found that two-thirds of adults believed their life would be over if they were diagnosed with dementia. So how do people adjust to the diagnosis and find ways of living with the condition? Understanding people's 'dementia representations' might tell us more about this and offer some ideas that could help people manage life with the condition.

In the MIDAS study, mentioned in Chapter 1, we had in-depth conversations with 64 people living with dementia about how they viewed the condition. Based on what they told us, we developed a set of questions that we could use to find out about people's 'dementia representations' (Quinn et al., 2018). We included these questions in our interviews with the IDEAL cohort participants at Time 1 (Clare et al., 2022). First, we checked whether people thought they were experiencing any changes or difficulties by asking about the typical effects of dementia. A few people, 7 in 100, did not think they had any difficulties; we did not ask people in this 'no problem' group any more questions. When we asked the rest what their condition was called, only one in four mentioned a diagnosis such as dementia or Alzheimer's. Instead, people talked about symptoms such as forgetfulness or memory loss, or commented on the distress that symptoms caused. When we specifically asked for a diagnosis, only one in two was able to tell us. When asked what caused the problem, the most common response was 'don't know', closely followed by 'brain changes' and 'ageing'.

One in three were unsure what would happen over time, with as many as one in five saying the condition would stay the same or improve. On a positive note, two out of three people thought there were things that could be done to help.

We looked for patterns in the way people answered the questions. We identified four groups each reflecting a particular kind of representation, plus the 'no problem' group (see Figure 2.2). People in the largest group, named 'symptoms' (49 per cent of the participants who answered the questions), talked about changes or difficulties rather than a diagnosis, thought these were due to brain changes or disease, and mostly believed things would get worse over time. The 'unclear' group (26 per cent) were unsure about the cause of their difficulties and expected these to stay the same over time. The 'diagnosis' group (14 per cent) used a medical term such as Alzheimer's to describe their difficulties, thought their condition was due to brain changes or disease, and mostly believed it would get worse over time. The 'ageing' group (11 per cent) talked about changes or difficulties rather than a diagnosis, and thought these changes were due to getting older.

We took the 'symptoms' group as our starting point for comparison with each of the other groups. The 'diagnosis' group tended to be younger and to have other health problems and had lower scores for living well. The 'ageing', 'unclear', and 'no problem' groups tended to do less well on cognitive tests but had higher scores for living well. People in the 'no problem' group had the highest living well scores of all. These differences stayed the same over the following two years.

Figure 2.2: Dementia representations among the IDEAL cohort.

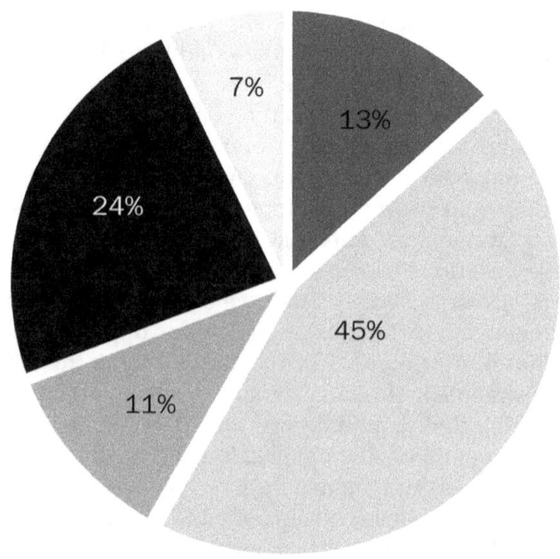

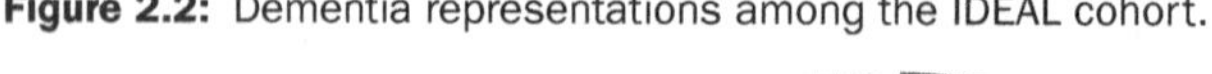

How people understood the condition was often quite different to the way in which medical experts think about it, and a significant number did not have a clear understanding. There could be several reasons why, for example, people thought the condition would stay the same or improve over time. Much of the information about dementia in the public domain, and the language and terminology used, is negative rather than simply factual or realistic. It is harder for all of us to remember information like this, which directly threatens our integrity (Cheston et al., 2018), especially as we get older, and many people with dementia experience memory difficulties. Equally, health professionals might not communicate information well, especially at difficult times such as when giving a diagnosis of dementia (Yates et al., 2021). The most important point, though, is that people who thought about dementia in a way that was different to medical experts tended to have better scores for living well than people who thought of the condition in the same way as medical experts. It seems their dementia representations made it easier for them to keep a sense of hope.

This is important for how we think and talk about dementia in public discourse, in fundraising and policy campaigns, and in health and social care services. How do we portray dementia realistically without being unduly negative? How can we balance a realistic portrayal of the condition that acknowledges the challenges it brings with the need for hope when living with, or caring for someone with, the condition?

In public discourse, the need to draw attention to the condition and secure funding can lead to a portrayal that emphasises challenges and burden. This is echoed and amplified in the media and shapes public understanding of dementia. It could be balanced by accounts reflecting the contributions people with dementia make, or the inventive strategies carers develop to get around problems. The evolution of new treatments for Alzheimer's disease, and in time perhaps also for other forms of dementia, will undoubtedly contribute to changing the way society views dementia. Encouraging a more proactive approach and promoting public debate on this issue would be timely.

For individuals, we need to rethink how we provide information about dementia, especially around the time of diagnosis, to allow people the chance to develop helpful ways of understanding and managing the condition. People are more likely to accept the diagnosis if it is communicated by a familiar and trusted health professional with time for discussion and follow-up. There are ways of providing information that can help make sure people take it in and remember key facts. Acknowledging the person's strengths and capabilities before presenting difficult or potentially distressing information makes it more likely the person will remember the details, and giving information in the form of examples helps people to engage with the content. Personal stories and accounts are helpful ways of conveying the idea that there is hope for people who are living with dementia. As people go on to adjust to life with the condition, understanding their dementia representations is key to supporting them in a way that matches their expectations. Many people will gain hope through linking with others who are also living with the condition, for example through in-person or online peer support groups, memory cafés and similar initiatives.

So what does this tell us about reconsidering living with dementia?

To rethink living with dementia, we must embrace diversity. Dementia is not one condition. Different types of dementia present different challenges for living with the condition, and these change as dementia progresses. People with dementia are not one single group. Dementia affects people from all walks of life and all kinds of backgrounds, with different beliefs, expectations, preferences, and living situations. The big picture provided by the IDEAL living well map offers a starting point for focusing on specific preferences and needs among individuals with dementia or among groups with different types of dementia or sharing certain characteristics, such as age or ethnicity. By doing this we can start to tackle disadvantage and make sure that everyone with dementia has an equal chance of getting the right support. This means putting the right structures in place on the one hand and changing attitudes on the other. To make this possible we need a shared understanding of dementia, a shared way of thinking and talking about dementia, that is realistic and yet offers hope for living with the condition.

Reflections from the ALWAYs group

This chapter really resonated with us. We are all different. We have different cultural backgrounds, tastes, and preferences. We may or may not have a carer, or have children, or be married, or live alone. Some of us identify as LGBTQ+. We have different dementia diagnoses, creating different challenges, so please don't assume that we all have Alzheimer's or that memory is our biggest problem. Start by finding out about us.

Key points

Key points for people with dementia and carers

- People can experience dementia very differently.
- There are different ways of thinking about dementia and what it means.
- Everyone has an equal right to good services and support.

Key points for health and social care practitioners

- Develop knowledge and understanding of rarer types of dementia.
- Challenge conscious or unconscious biases that might influence access to your services.
- Try to understand people's dementia representations and tailor your approach accordingly.

> **Key points for policy-makers**
>
> - Distinguish between different types and stages of dementia.
> - Promote equitable access to services and work to build trust.
> - Portray dementia realistically while offering hope that people can live well
>   with the condition.

 **Manifesto statement**

We are all different: we want you to find out about us so you can best enable
us to live with dementia.

References

Cahill, S. and Diaz-Ponce, A. (2011) 'I hate having nobody here. I'd like to know where
they all are': can qualitative research detect differences in quality of life among nursing home residents with different levels of cognitive impairment?, *Aging and Mental
Health*, 15(5): 562–72.

Cheston, R., Dodd, E., Christopher, G., Jones, C., Wildschut, T., & Sedikides, C. (2018)
Selective forgetting of self-threatening statements: mnemic neglect for dementia
information in people with mild dementia. *International Journal of Geriatric Psychiatry*, 33(8), 1065–1073. Available at: https://doi.org/10.1002/gps.4894

Clare, L., Rowlands, J., Bruce, E., et al. (2008) The experience of living with dementia
in residential care: an interpretative phenomenological analysis, *The Gerontologist*,
48(6): 711–20.

Clare, L., Martyr, A., Henderson, C., et al. (2020) Living alone with mild-to-moderate
dementia: findings from the IDEAL cohort, *Journal of Alzheimer's Disease*, 78(3):
1207–16.

Clare, L., Gamble, L.D., Martyr, A., et al. (2022) Psychological processes in adapting to
dementia: illness representations among the IDEAL cohort, *Psychology and Aging*,
37(4): 524–41.

Clare, L., Gamble, L.D., Martyr, A., et al. (2024) Living alone with mild-to-moderate
dementia over a two-year period: longitudinal findings from the IDEAL cohort, *American Journal of Geriatric Psychiatry*, 32(11): 1309–21.

Gamble, L.D., Matthews, F.E., Jones, I.R., et al. (2022) Characteristics of people living
with undiagnosed dementia: findings from the CFAS-Wales study, *BMC Geriatrics*,
22(1): 409. Available at: https://doi.org/10.1186/s12877-022-03086-4.

Hagger, M.S. and Orbell, S. (2022) The common sense model of illness self-regulation: a
conceptual review and proposed extended model, *Health Psychology Review*, 16(3):
347–77.

Henderson, C., Knapp, M., Nelis, S.M., et al. (2019) Use and costs of services and unpaid
care for people with mild-to-moderate dementia: baseline results from the IDEAL
cohort study, *Alzheimer's and Dementia: Translational Research and Clinical
Interventions*, 5(1): 685–96.

Henderson, C., Knapp, M., Martyr, A., et al. (2022) The use and costs of paid and unpaid care for people with dementia: findings from three waves of the IDEAL cohort programme, *Journal of Alzheimer's Disease*, 86(1): 135–53.

Henley, J., Hillman, A., Jones, I.R., et al. (2021) 'We're happy as we are': the experience of living with possible undiagnosed dementia, *Ageing and Society*, 43(9): 2041–66.

Martyr, A., Gamble, L.D., Hunt, A., et al. (2024) Differences in trajectories of quality of life according to type of dementia: 6-year longitudinal findings from the IDEAL programme, *BMC Medicine*, 22(1): 265. Available at: https://doi.org/10.1186/s12916-024-03492-y.

Mayhew, P.A., Acton, G.J., Yauk, S., et al. (2001) Communication from individuals with advanced DAT: can it provide clues to their sense of self-awareness and well-being?, *Geriatric Nursing*, 22(2): 108–10.

National Institute for Health and Care Excellence (NICE) (2018) *Dementia: Assessment, management and support for people living with dementia and their carers*, NICE Guideline NG97. Available at: https://www.nice.org.uk/guidance/ng97 (accessed 10 September 2024).

Quinn, C., Morris, R.G. and Clare, L. (2018) Beliefs about dementia: development and validation of the Representations and Adjustment to Dementia Index (RADIX), *American Journal of Geriatric Psychiatry*, 26(6): 680–89.

Sabatini, S., Martyr, A., Gamble, L.D., et al. (2024) Identifying predictors of transition to a care home for people with dementia: findings from the IDEAL programme, *Aging and Mental Health*. Available at: https://doi.org/10.1080/13607863.2024.2383367.

van Horik, J.O., Collins, R., Martyr, A., et al. (2022) Limited receipt of support services among people with mild-to-moderate dementia: findings from the IDEAL cohort, *International Journal of Geriatric Psychiatry*, 37(3): e5688. Available at: https://doi.org/10.1002/gps.5688.

Victor, C., Gamble, L.D., Pentecost, C., et al. (2024a) Living well with dementia: an exploratory matched analysis of minority ethnic and white people with dementia and carers participating in the IDEAL programme, *International Journal of Geriatric Psychiatry*, 39(1): e6048. Available at: https://doi.org/10.1002/gps.6048.

Victor, C., van den Heuvel, E., Pentecost, C., et al. (2024b) Perspectives of minority ethnic caregivers of people with dementia interviewed as part of the IDEAL programme, *Health and Social Care in the Community*. Available at: https://doi.org/10.1155/2024/8732644.

World Health Organization (WHO) (2017) *Global Action Plan on Dementia*. Available at: https://www.who.int/publications/i/item/global-action-plan-on-the-public-health-response-to-dementia-2017–2025 (accessed 2 August 2024).

Wu, Y.-T., Clare, L., Hindle, J.V., et al. (2018) Dementia subtype and living well: results from the Improving the experience of Dementia and Enhancing Active Life (IDEAL) study, *BMC Medicine*, 16(1): 140. Available at: https://doi.org/10.1186/s12916-018-1135-2.

Yates, J., Stanyon, M., Samra, R., et al. (2021) Challenges in disclosing and receiving a diagnosis of dementia: a systematic review of practice from the perspectives of people with dementia, carers, and healthcare professionals, *International Psychogeriatrics*, 33(11): 1161–92.

3

How can you 'live well' with dementia?

Catherine Charlwood

> *Being happy, or at least content with my physical and mental capabilities …*
> *To be as independent as my condition will allow.*
>
> (An IDEAL participant living with dementia)

In this chapter we will:

- discuss the origins of the phrase 'living well with dementia'
- reveal how people with dementia and those supporting them understand this phrase
- demonstrate the variety of meanings 'living well' holds
- introduce co-produced resources to help people live life as they choose

Life writ large

Can you remember how you felt when you first heard the phrase 'living well with dementia'? Did you raise your eyebrows? You are not alone: it is a fair response, and one which deserves consideration.

We have heard about the range of different things that influence the experience of living with dementia. Only certain features of the broader picture will be relevant for each individual. Adapting support services to this is called 'personalisation', and personalisation is an important aim for health and social care: it both benefits people and means that services are used more efficiently, which is vital given that resources are always limited. While previous chapters looked at the IDEAL cohort as a whole, the focus now turns to the experience of dementia on an individual basis: experiences of dementia are deeply personal. However, everyone's experience is lived within the context of structural frameworks, such as medical referrals, the welfare system, and what certain funds may be used for, or simply which services exist in their area. Personal experience may or may not fit well within these structures.

'Living well' has life at its heart and, like life, 'living well' with dementia is complex, individual, and prone to change. This chapter, then, expands how we think about dementia, to understand it within the broad sweep of things – good and bad – that each individual life embraces. Living well with dementia depends on much more than diagnosis or treatment: this is life writ large.

Where does 'living well' come from?

We focus primarily on an English or UK context because IDEAL was based in Great Britain. However, this is also where the phrase first came to prominence. 'Living well with dementia: A national dementia strategy' was published in 2009 to outline a vision of an England where 'all people with dementia and their carers should live well with dementia' (Department of Health, 2009: 7). It emerged against a backdrop of very negative views of dementia, discussed below. Although the phrase now proliferates through strategies large and small, and can be found on numerous websites and materials, it sprang into awareness with the launch of the national strategy.

A review of national dementia strategies across Europe identified receiving a timely diagnosis as a common theme 'to allow for effective treatment and interventions, to allow the person to plan for the future and to ensure services and supports can be put in place to help the person live well with the condition for as long as possible' (Alzheimer Europe, 2018: 17). Like England, Austria elected to title their 2015 strategy 'Living well with dementia'. While the development of these national strategies saw a considerable consultation process, including with people with dementia and carers, the eventual documents are necessarily phrased in the language of health policy (Banerjee, 2010). In these strategies, living well with dementia is something to be achieved by systems and large organisations reaching certain objectives. This is at a remove from the individual lives which may, or may not, be lived well with dementia – either in their own estimation, or by that of an aspirational strategy.

The UK 'Prime Minister's challenge on dementia 2020' declared its ambition for England to be 'the best country in the world for dementia care and support and for people with dementia, their carers and families to live' (Department of Health, 2015: 3). As part of the implementation plan, the NHS launched 'The Well Pathway for Dementia': preventing well, diagnosing well, supporting well, living well, and dying well. 'Living well' is defined broadly: 'People with dementia can live normally in safe and accepting communities' (NHS England, 2016). This alludes to stigma as part of life with dementia, though carers are absent from this definition, whereas the preceding 'supporting well' seeks to assure 'Access to safe high quality health & social care for people with dementia and carers'. 'Living well' can, depending on other health conditions and time since diagnosis, account for a significant number of years within this pathway. However, again this is the terminology of an organisation. Furthermore, we know that many people living with dementia and those supporting them receive little support from formal health and care services (see Chapter 10). 'Living well with dementia', then, seems to have developed top-down from authoritative voices: those in power rather than those affected by the condition. Although now widely used, this phrase seems to be driven more by professionals and organisations than individuals affected by dementia.

A contested phrase

One carer told us, *'There is no such thing as "living well with dementia", there is only coping with dementia'*. The term 'living well' is, understandably, not universally liked. Some people feel that it sets too high a bar or makes it the fault of the individual if they 'fail' to 'live well'. Others think it is an unreasonable term to use alongside a progressive and ultimately terminal condition like dementia. Certainly, there are days when living well is difficult or impossible, but there are also better days. Knowing what makes better days better, and how to harness that, is important for us all.

As Keith from the ALWAYs group noted, *'It's about ownership of the phrase "living well" – who owns that phrase? Can we take it back?'*. This highlights the issue of control: who controls public discourse and, therefore, has the power to shape circumstances for others. Considering 'living well with dementia' should be seen as an opportunity to get to know that individual and understand what matters to them to both maintain what is working well and improve their life.

Dementia advocate Wendy Mitchell contested the phrase in a book section entitled 'On language used by professionals', remarking:

> I prefer 'living as well as your circumstances allow' so people don't feel inadequate when they're struggling, and that is something that everyone can aim for, whatever their personal or financial situation. It's also open to interpretation because the idea of 'living well' for one person is not the same for another … It comes with less pressure, less fear of failure, fewer impossible dreams to achieve.
>
> (Mitchell, 2022: 97–98)

Crucially, as Mitchell says, what constitutes living well differs for each individual. Not only have we researched this in IDEAL, but we have created resources specifically to encourage practitioners and professionals to delve into the meaning it holds for the individual in front of them, so that they can best support that person.

Living well with dementia does not mean that everything is constantly going well. That is an unrealistic goal for anyone, and perhaps especially for people living with dementia and their families. When we discussed this with the ALWAYs group, they were keen to point out that consistent good days are unnatural: living well includes harder days where things are more of a struggle. Indeed, Jacqui pointed out that *'it's annoying if people are always trying to make you happy!'*.

You might wonder why the phrase 'living well' is sometimes in inverted commas. This is to indicate that it is a concept, an idea that covers many things. The IDEAL definition of 'living well' may not be the same as other people's, or yours:

> We use 'living well' here in the sense that people experiencing the challenges of living with dementia can and should be enabled to experience the best achievable state of health and subjective well-being, acknowledging that this requires a facilitative social and environmental context and appropriate support.
>
> (Clare et al., 2023: 2)

Our definition of living well goes beyond a narrow focus on symptoms. IDEAL has evolved since 2014, as have understandings of dementia in society at large. We no longer tend to talk about 'living well' with dementia, but instead we talk about living with dementia or living as you choose with dementia. Dementia is a condition with which people live, but the focus is on the living: life is still there to be lived, albeit with adjustments and adaptations. As the ALWAYs group would point out, the *living* is more important than the dementia when we say 'living with dementia'. In this, we extend Kitwood's insistence that the 'frame of reference should no longer be person-with-DEMENTIA, but PERSON-with-dementia' (Kitwood, 1997: 7). Kitwood's focus was on retaining personhood, emphasising this by the noun 'person' remaining constant. In line with some changes in perception and the IDEAL intention of 'enhancing active life', we focus on 'living' – the dynamic verb which must remain dynamic.

Is 'living well with dementia' a useful phrase? To answer this, we might consider whether the alternative is useful. The 2024 World Alzheimer Report revealed how worried people are globally about dementia: the proportions of the public who think people with dementia are 'dangerous' (29–32 per cent) or 'impulsive and unpredictable' (64 per cent) have both increased. Meanwhile, people with dementia and carers report discrimination and avoidance of social activities and public interactions for fear of judgement or mistreatment (Alzheimer's Disease International, 2024: 9–10). In the UK, the 2023 Dementia Attitudes Monitor found that almost half of the 2,522 people asked agreed with the statement 'Dementia is the health condition I fear most about getting in the future' (Alzheimer's Research UK, 2023: 21). When dementia is feared, stigma thrives: people are less likely to come forward for diagnosis, or to have a good quality of life with dementia.

This is not about creating false hope – indeed, our conversations have revolved around realistic hope: what can realistically be hoped for when living with dementia – but about keeping the possibility of positivity in play. This matters because negative feelings influence a person's ability to feel that they are living well (see Chapter 9). While it is important to acknowledge the many challenges dementia brings and mitigate them as best we can, it is also important not to write people off when a dementia diagnosis enters the scene.

The introduction emphasised the importance of the language we use around dementia. A linguistics project, Public Discourses of Dementia, recently investigated this. Analysing the metaphors used about dementia in 6,751 tabloid newspaper articles revealed a pattern of negativity:

> Dementia stigma is, I would argue, propagated not only through the use of violence metaphors but also by other metaphorical framings identified here, including those of horrors and nightmares … These tropes foreground dementia's most disastrous and fear-inducing aspects while backgrounding, if not shutting down altogether, the possibility of 'living well' with dementia.
>
> (Brookes, 2023: 225)

Whether you personally find 'living well with dementia' a useful phrase or not, this fearmongering is not useful either to people currently experiencing dementia, or those who will go on to do so. It is important to keep our shared humanity in view. As Kitwood asserts, we need to enable 'men and women with dementia [to continue] to live in the world of persons, and not being downgraded into the carriers of an organic brain disease' (1997: 7).

What did people with dementia say?

We asked IDEAL participants 'What does living well mean to you?'; 1,339 people living with dementia answered the question, asked at Time 1. This alone gives you a sense of the range of responses IDEAL gathered. This response from one participant shows how some people defined 'living well' expansively: *'Living well is relative to my current situation … Living well is about meeting competing demands of what I want to do, what I can do, and taking part in family life'* (Quinn et al., 2022: 3).

We wanted to understand whether people's own ideas about living well resonated with the domains of experience research suggested influenced people's lives. We grouped similar answers together into ten categories (see Figure 3.1). These mapped onto what we found from the questionnaires people completed, confirming that we should be thinking about all these aspects of people's lives.

Some people felt they were not living well. However, some of the reasons people identified, such as loss of independence, are things that could be partially restored with appropriate support. This 'demonstrates that a person's capability to live well is not purely determined by the impact the diagnosis of dementia is having on that person's life' (Quinn et al., 2022: 4). Building up a picture of how people living with dementia understand this phrase presents new opportunities:

- Seeing how important it is to consider the whole person and what may be affecting their well-being.
- Identifying the things that influence a person's ability to live well which are modifiable, through policy changes, social initiatives, and support from services and community sources.

Enabling people to live well with dementia requires a broad approach: this includes both health and social care systems and the wider community.

It takes more than one: living well together

The networks surrounding a person living with dementia are crucial. As Figure 3.1 shows, almost half the answers to 'What does living well mean to you?' pertained to relationships. While I focus here on the perspective of the person as the nucleus of a broader network, later chapters consider carers and connections with the wider community.

Many people participating in IDEAL also had a carer participate with them. A person with dementia and the person supporting them form an important

Figure 3.1: Responses to the question 'What does living well mean to you?'.

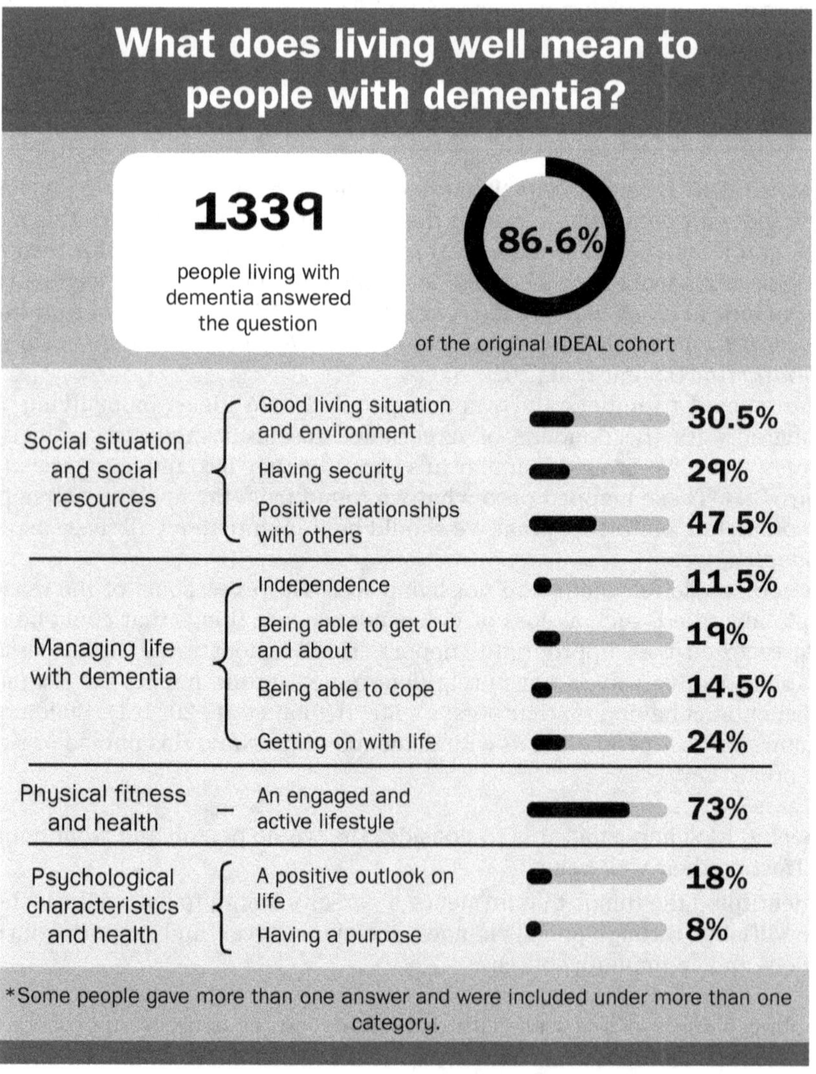

unit, and how they feel about their individual lives affects both. We asked carers the same question, and one of the most striking things when looking at their responses is the number of times carers answered with reference to the person with dementia they were supporting. This reinforces the fact that when a carer is involved, the needs of both persons must be considered together.

My play on 'it takes two' in the heading above is purposeful: it takes everyone's involvement to improve the experience of living with dementia, from family members to café staff, to the impatient shopper behind a person with dementia determinedly facing the seeming conundrum of the cashpoint. We knew that we needed to create not only resources for individuals themselves, but also resources that focused on these wider networks, so that people affected by dementia live within communities that are understanding and environments that are adaptive. Here, I introduce the resources we co-produced for different purposes.

Exploring whether people are living well

As mentioned, there was no direct way of measuring whether anyone was living well. Pre-existing questionnaires measured similar things, such as quality of life or well-being, but many were developed for research purposes, so tended to be lengthy and complex, and were not necessarily designed with and for people with dementia. Building on the data, IDEAL researchers set about co-producing a new questionnaire: the My Life Questionnaire.

Over a period of four years, we worked with a co-production group of people living with dementia to develop a questionnaire that 'people would want to fill in', as Chris, one of the members, put it. This meant it should be accessible, short, have only a few options to choose from, focus on the here and now, and use positive wording. The group named itself the Dementia Experts into Action Research (DEAR) group; some members participated throughout, and others joined or left. The group came to the view that 'the questionnaire should focus on how people perceive their life while living with dementia, rather than on the experience of dementia itself' (Clare et al., 2023: 7). This is probably why it contains no specific references to dementia or its symptoms.

The questionnaire consists of statements that people can agree with or disagree with. These were developed from responses to the question 'What does living well mean to you?'. An initial set of 230 statements was gradually reduced to a long-list of 41. These were tested to determine whether the statements were easy to answer, whether people found them acceptable, and whether they gave us useful information. Fifty-three people with dementia responded to the statements. Based on both statistical analyses and the views of co-production group members, we selected 12 statements to test further in the next round of data collection. Our analyses showed that 10 of the statements both worked well and covered a range of aspects of everyday life. We looked in more detail at this set of 10 statements to see whether the scores across the 10 statements suggested that, taken together, they were capturing something meaningful about living well. We compared the way people responded with how they scored on other relevant questionnaires. The pattern of scores fitted well with what we expected. For example, the results were similar enough to research questionnaires measuring quality of life and well-being to give us confidence, but different enough for this new questionnaire to be useful. The 10 statements therefore formed the final version of the questionnaire (see Figure 3.2).

Figure 3.2: The My Life Questionnaire.

My Life Questionnaire

This questionnaire is about your daily life. We hope that, as you look over your answers, you can see which areas are going well for you. You might also identify areas where you or others could make changes to improve how you feel about your life. You might want to discuss your answers with your family, friends or health and care professionals.

Filling in the questionnaire

Over the page are 10 statements about daily life. For each statement, please choose the response that best matches how you feel. These are the responses you can choose from:

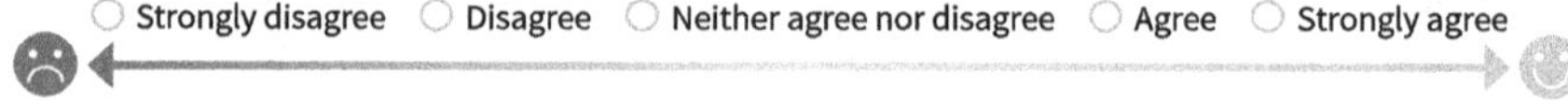

You can respond to the statements in any order.

If you feel emotional as you complete the questionnaire, you could take a look at the Living with Dementia Toolkit. It is full of support, ideas, and inspiration from people with dementia:
www.livingwithdementiatoolkit.org.uk

Scoring the questionnaire

You score the questionnaire as follows:

1 Award points for each statement:
- Strongly disagree = **1**
- Disagree = **2**
- Neither agree nor disagree = **3**
- Agree = **4**
- Strongly agree = **5**

2 Add up the points for **all 10 items to get the score.**

3 The **minimum** possible score is **10**. The **maximum** possible score is **50**.

The My Life Questionnaire has been co-produced by people living with dementia and the IDEAL research team, and scientifically validated as part of the IDEAL research programme.

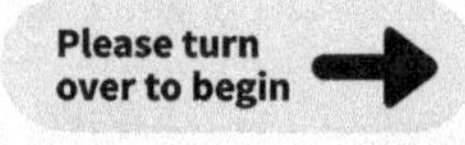

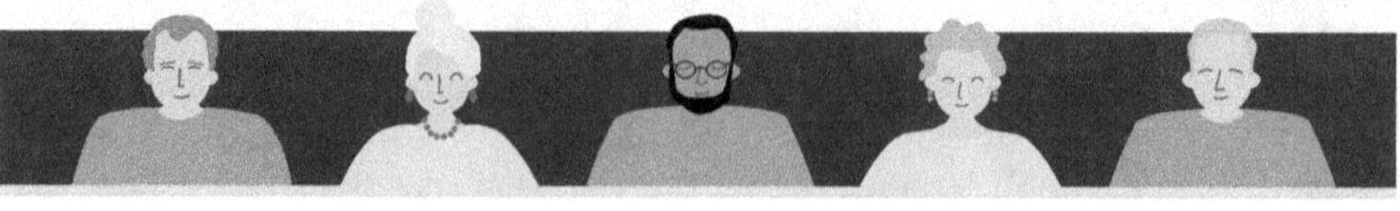

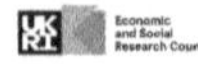

(Continued)

Figure 3.2: (*Continued*)

My Life Questionnaire

○ Strongly disagree   ○ Disagree   ○ Neither agree nor disagree   ○ Agree   ○ Strongly agree

I keep my mind occupied
○ Strongly disagree   ○ Disagree   ○ Neither agree nor disagree   ○ Agree   ○ Strongly agree

I have people to talk to
○ Strongly disagree   ○ Disagree   ○ Neither agree nor disagree   ○ Agree   ○ Strongly agree

I usually sleep well
○ Strongly disagree   ○ Disagree   ○ Neither agree nor disagree   ○ Agree   ○ Strongly agree

I like where I live
○ Strongly disagree   ○ Disagree   ○ Neither agree nor disagree   ○ Agree   ○ Strongly agree

I am able to stay active
○ Strongly disagree   ○ Disagree   ○ Neither agree nor disagree   ○ Agree   ○ Strongly agree

I spend time with friends
○ Strongly disagree   ○ Disagree   ○ Neither agree nor disagree   ○ Agree   ○ Strongly agree

I am able to relax
○ Strongly disagree   ○ Disagree   ○ Neither agree nor disagree   ○ Agree   ○ Strongly agree

I can get out and about when I want to
○ Strongly disagree   ○ Disagree   ○ Neither agree nor disagree   ○ Agree   ○ Strongly agree

I feel useful
○ Strongly disagree   ○ Disagree   ○ Neither agree nor disagree   ○ Agree   ○ Strongly agree

I have someone I can call on in an emergency
○ Strongly disagree   ○ Disagree   ○ Neither agree nor disagree   ○ Agree   ○ Strongly agree

The co-production group helped to prepare an initial design brief and then had a back-and-forth dialogue with the designer to find a way of presenting the questionnaire that was as accessible and appealing as possible. They asked that the instructions include something regarding what to do if you felt emotional while completing the questionnaire. The group members also helped rationalise the final order of the statements: they were adamant that 'I feel useful' was the most important and should be near the end. They did not want 'I am able to stay active' to come too early, because if you are inactive for reasons other than dementia, that could make you unhappy and colour how you approach the other questions.

The final questionnaire is a true marriage of research evidence and real-life experience. The My Life Questionnaire is freely available for anyone to use via the 'How are you feeling today?' page of the Living with Dementia Toolkit (IDEAL Programme, 2021). This questionnaire provides a snapshot of how someone is doing. Completing it again after a gap could help to track whether and how things are changing. If widely adopted – in large surveys, for example – it could also tell us how people with dementia are doing as a group.

The My Life Questionnaire is a standardised questionnaire meaning that everyone answers the same questions. However, for individuals to live their version of a good life, they might want to keep track of how they are doing in relation to activities of their choosing. The co-production group later helped IDEAL develop My Life Today, a personalised tracker that allows people living with dementia to identify the things which bring them joy, consider whether they are experiencing these things or doing them enough, and if not, think about how to incorporate them better. The group helped develop the tool, agree the design and content, and prepare the accompanying information and illustrative examples. My Life Today was tested with 16 people with dementia and 4 supporters (Pentecost et al., 2024). People found it a useful tool to help keep preferred activities in view, and resourcefully identified ways of using it that best suited their needs. My Life Today is now freely available to download from www.idealproject.org.uk/projects/mylifetoday.

Promoting 'living well' in different ways

People with dementia can do a lot to enable themselves to live with the condition, and often want that opportunity, but they also need and benefit from support. During the COVID-19 pandemic, social contacts were limited and while looking at how people with dementia were affected, we also thought about what support might be helpful. This led to the idea of a toolkit specifically to help people through the period of social restrictions. However, it evolved into a long-lasting and comprehensive resource which draws on the breadth of IDEAL findings: it became the Living with Dementia Toolkit (Figure 3.3).

We grouped resources under five key themes: Stay safe and well; Stay connected; Keep a sense of purpose; Stay active; and Stay positive. These themes

Figure 3.3: The Living with Dementia Toolkit logo.

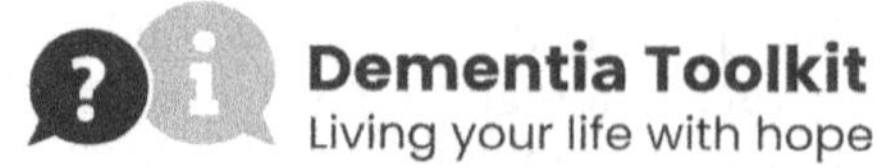

map onto the domains that we found were related to being able to 'live well' in the IDEAL research. We formed a co-production group consisting of four people living with dementia, four carers, a group facilitator, and myself. We met fortnightly to discuss ideas, co-produce the design, and more.

While there were topics we always knew we would cover from our research, through our co-production discussions new topics emerged as significant. People with dementia and carers kept mentioning risk, but had differing views about it: 'Carers are often focused on reducing risks, usually for good reasons. But this can result in people with dementia feeling disempowered' (Batchelor et al., 2023: 23). Our discussions eventually became the 'Rethinking risk' resource. In having these conversations, we had to listen to different opinions and find a way to reach consensus. As Chris said, 'being wrapped in cotton wool can be as disabling as dementia', and Jacqui emphasised that 'The impact of criticizing people with dementia can be huge. It knocks your confidence and makes you not want to try again' (Batchelor et al., 2023: 23).

The variety of resources included in the Living with Dementia Toolkit is intentional. Similarly, there is a range of media: text, pictures, video and audio. Not everything will appeal to everybody, but they can pick and choose what suits them. The aim is to offer people with dementia and carers:

- hope for the future
- examples of real-life experiences
- ideas to help you live your life as you choose

While the fullest experience is found online, we also created a printable guide and PDF versions of each resource. Rather than being prescriptive, the Toolkit invites individuals to explore *what* they want to *when* they want to. Distributed widely across NHS Trusts, national third sector organisations, and by individuals attending or facilitating their local groups, the Living with Dementia Toolkit is a hopeful resource that focuses on living. Internationally, it has had visitors from over 150 countries and is part of the WHO's Global Dementia Observatory Knowledge Exchange Forum.

We should also remember the support provided by friends, who can enable the continued agency and independence of a person with dementia. A specially commissioned song, 'Brave New World', written and performed by two men living with dementia, incites the listener to act: 'it's a new world – so go out and find it' (Thred CIC, 2022). While it offers people living with dementia agency to act for themselves, they are not expected to do this alone: 'Look at your life and all you give, / We all stand beside you so you can live, / In your new world'.

The song takes its title from Shakespeare's *The Tempest*: Miranda marvels in wonder at the people she suddenly encounters, having been starved of human company. This same phrase inspired Aldous Huxley's dystopian novel, so 'brave new world' already symbolises both the good and the bad. The song was written by two men in Liverpool, Paul and Tommy, both of whom are also co-directors of Thred CIC, a regional organisation supporting people living with dementia. A big part of the way Paul and Tommy live with dementia is through their deep friendship and shared love of music. We commissioned them to write a song for IDEAL, having heard their music online and been moved by their honest but hopeful attitude towards dementia. We shared some of the findings with them and this was the message they took forward. 'Brave New World' has had over 2,700 plays on YouTube and became the official song of the 35th Global Alzheimer's Disease International Conference in London, 2022, played after keynote talks and panel sessions.

Resources to promote public awareness

How people with dementia experience their lives is in part shaped by the environments they live in and the networks and communities surrounding them. To change things for the better, we need to involve the broader public in understanding dementia. Over the course of IDEAL, we have incorporated different arts-based projects for this purpose.

In collaboration with artist and photographer Ian Beesley, cartoonist Tony Husband, poet Ian McMillan, and designer Martyn Hall, the 'A Life More Ordinary' project aimed to document what it is like to live with dementia. Through a series of workshops, dementia peer support groups in English towns created chapbooks which focused on their chosen interests. The Budding Friends group in Exeter produced 'The Allotment of Time', documenting their shared present working on their allotment, as well as precious photographs and memories from group members' individual pasts. One of these groups, made up of members from three peer support groups in Yorkshire, chose to focus their chapbook on accessibility of public transport and the barriers to enjoying 'A Grand Day Out'. Then they had an idea. How about making a banner that would really cause people to sit up and take notice? They worked with the artists to create a large double-sided banner in the style of a trade union banner, with one side showing the barriers and challenges, and the other the benefits, of 'A Grand Day Out'. They arranged for the banner to be unfurled in public at York Railway Station, accompanied by a brass band (typical of the area) and with press and photographers invited, as shown in the photograph on the following page.

This initiative inspired other groups to follow suit, and 'A Life More Ordinary' evolved into 'The Unfurlings: Banners for Hope and Change'. Sixteen groups across the country worked with the artists to create their own banners. Themes included user-friendliness of technology such as cash points, accessibility of health and care services, inclusion of people from minority ethnic groups, and the importance of friendship. The full set of banners was exhibited at the People's History Museum in Manchester in December 2019, and then toured various venues in England. They were also published in a book (Beesley et al., 2020) and put in context by an insightful essay on the history of banners authored by Professor Selina Todd. The banners were an effective and enjoyable way to highlight the changes which need to occur to enable people living with dementia to continue leading full lives within the community.

The unfurling of the Yorkshire DEEP banner at York Railway Station.

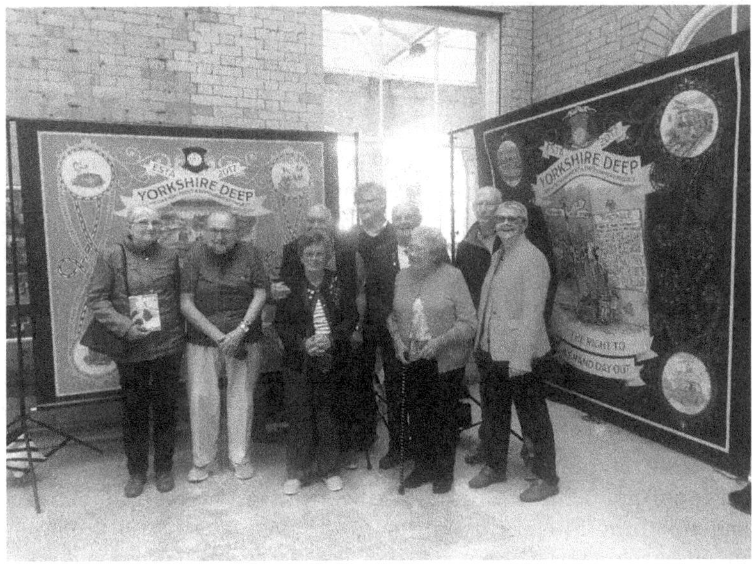

Drama offered another route to encouraging public awareness and debate about how dementia is understood. In collaboration with theatre director Paul Jepson, we decided to focus on communication. Our ALWAYs group helped to select different scenarios from real life where there can be a 'tipping point' in communication between a person with dementia and the family member, friend, or professional they are talking to. We used a forum theatre method, staging scenarios and then inviting the audience to respond and suggest ways in which the interaction could play out differently, leading to a more constructive outcome. This method demonstrates how the eventual outcome is shaped by the way in which people communicate with each other: the same event could end in confusion and anger or in understanding and reduced stress. This empowers viewers to think about their own approach and, perhaps, to try reacting in a different way.

Paul worked with the actors to develop the scenarios, taking advice from the ALWAYs group, and to explore in rehearsal the various ways in which they could play out. The resulting live play, consisting of five scenarios, was called 'The World Turned Upside Down'. Scenarios were improvised one way, and then Paul asked the audience to comment on what they had seen. Based on audience feedback, the same scenario was replayed for a different outcome. We filmed the rehearsals, creation process, performances, and reflections on the project to create a documentary film of the same name, which is freely available on YouTube. The film version of 'The World Turned Upside Down' explores what we could do differently and how to communicate better. Beyond thousands of views online, the film has been used in public screenings to promote discussion of dementia and individual scenarios are being used for educational purposes, such as the 'doctor's appointment' scenario being used in training medical students.

Fuelled by the success of the play and film, we applied to the Arts Council of Wales for funding for 'Living with dementia: An operatic exploration to promote understanding and reduce stigma'. At the heart of the project was the creation of a new one-act opera, 'The Bridge', centring on a man's experience of the journey from noticing something is wrong to being diagnosed and experiencing well-intentioned – if sometimes misguided – attempts to help him, demonstrating the emotional and practical challenges of adjusting to a dementia diagnosis. The libretto was developed by director Marian Bryfdir and the score by composer Edward Wright. Alongside the opera, we also ran community workshops to find out how people felt dementia was supported, or not, within their local communities.

All three of these projects proved the value of sharing our work with the public. An older teenager in the audience of 'The World Turned Upside Down' play noted, 'I thought [dementia] was an illness where it just kind of snaps on and it's very simple, but it's a long process, which I hadn't noticed before' (IDEAL Programme, 2022: 1:16:48). We were also humbled by the reactions from seasoned practitioners: even those who deal with these situations daily were moved to tears by the opera.

Arts-based work reaches people in new ways. Its subjective nature allows audiences to find their own personal relationship with what is presented. We must not underestimate the importance of involving broader publics in discussions about dementia, as dementia affects us all, and the experience of dementia is affected by each person's behaviour.

'With appropriate support': what it takes to live well

I often find myself writing or saying the caveat 'with appropriate support' (or similar): with appropriate support, people can live well with dementia. As a government report notes, 'with early intervention, and access to the right services and support, people with dementia can continue to live well for many years' (Department of Health, 2013: 14). This phrasing can sound long-winded: it is tempting to leave it out. When 'living well with dementia' is quoted by itself, it sounds like something that people are supposed to manifest by willpower alone and this risks 'living well' leaning towards meaning individual responsibility (Bartlett et al., 2017). Therefore, the 'with appropriate support' aspect of living well cannot remain implicit.

Living life as you choose is not something which rests on the shoulders of people with dementia and those supporting them to achieve alone. Living what you personally consider to be a good life with dementia can be enabled, or frustrated, by external circumstances and the systems surrounding you. As the ALWAYs group kept reminding us, '*it's all very well talking about living well but if it takes money and some people don't have that, then we're excluding people*'. Quite right.

Chapter 10 looks at the role of services and support, but here I turn attention to how carers participating in IDEAL responded when asked, 'What do you think could be done by the government to help people live well with dementia?'. Calls for research and increased knowledge and understanding were strongly represented among the 832 responses, but there was a particular emphasis on economic aspects. Words relating to finances had 358 mentions, with 'help' and 'support' – both of which inevitably come with a bill for someone to foot – seeing 407 mentions. What is clear in reading these answers is the need for funding to be available to help people right now, as well as preparing for future funding needs.

I have emphasised individual differences in the experience of dementia, and this is true economically as well. As one carer wrote, '*We made plans for pension etc. for our 60s. We are in our 50s now with savings for our retirement at 65 so what happens for 15 years? No one seems to know that exceptions need to be made*'. Young-onset dementia poses different financial challenges.

In writing this, I've come to a greater respect of the conjunction 'with'. This seemingly inconsequential word is, in fact, at the heart of the experience of 'living well with dementia'. 'With' has many meanings. Most obviously, 'with' introduces the condition which necessarily shapes what is possible in terms of living well: dementia provides a significant new overlay to the experience of life. 'With' also suggests the additions which come alongside dementia – the adaptations and modifications necessary to continue your chosen activities – be that a Blue Badge which enables you to park in disabled spaces in the UK, building in an extra 30 minutes to get ready to go out, or having Alexa poised to give an appointment reminder. I also read a sense of togetherness in the 'with' of 'living well with dementia'. We always intended to look at not just individuals, but relationships and communities of a range of sizes. Dementia is never experienced alone – all kinds of people are met along the way in planned and accidental encounters – so each one of us has a role to play in shaping the experience of dementia.

So what does this tell us about reconsidering dementia?

Dementia care research like IDEAL is founded on the belief that action can and should be taken to improve the lives of people with dementia and those supporting them. This should not be a radical proposition. Indeed, it is not a belief but a fact that actions can always be taken to improve quality of life: that difference – however small – might have a huge impact.

We began by looking at pre-constructed frameworks into which individual experiences of dementia are asked to fit. This tends to result in neither the best support nor the best care, because each person's experience is individual. In IDEAL, we have mapped, as thoroughly as possible, the broad picture of all the things which influence the experience of dementia. This is not to provide another framework to fit to, but so that we can begin from a position of thinking inclusively about dementia without pre-judging what affects this person, or indeed what interests them. Our co-produced resources, then, enable the individual, or a practitioner or professional, to overlay their unique set of experiences onto that broader map: we have drawn the night sky so that individual constellations can be seen within it.

Reflections from the ALWAYs group

Some of us personally do not like the phrase 'living well with dementia'. We no longer use it to discuss dementia. However, we could see the arguments for its usage and think it is useful to have this described. Understanding the history of this phrase is essential. We think that this chapter should challenge the readers to think about this phrase and what it means.

We thought the 'Living well together' section was very important. 'Living well with dementia' is so very related to both how well the networks of a person with dementia are able to adjust to changes following a diagnosis and how well services work for each individual. Those networks could include a carer, family, friends – never forget that how people surrounding the person with dementia live with the diagnosis can really affect the person.

Key points

Key points for people with dementia and carers

- Your life with dementia is yours to define.
- There are ways of improving your life with dementia and you have a right to support.
- Finding living with dementia hard is natural: you are allowed to struggle and are encouraged to seek help as you need.

Key points for health and social care practitioners

- Co-produced resources which reflect the voices of people affected by dementia are freely available: use and promote them.
- Think about the whole person when planning how to support an individual.
- Ask people what they want, don't tell them what they need.

Key points for policy-makers

- Policy planning requires a personalised, rather than one-size-fits-all, approach.
- Policy decisions about living with dementia must take account of the views of those living the reality.
- Realistic and suitable financial and instrumental support for families affected by dementia is crucial to living well.

 **Manifesto statement**

We want to live in a way that suits us and be supported to adapt to changes.

References

Alzheimer Europe (2018) *Dementia in Europe Yearbook 2018: Comparison of national dementia strategies in Europe.* Luxembourg: Alzheimer Europe. Available at: https://www.alzheimer-europe.org/sites/default/files/alzheimer_europe_dementia_in_europe_yearbook_2018.pdf.

Alzheimer's Disease International (2024) *World Alzheimer Report 2024: Changes to attitudes in dementia.* London: Alzheimer's Disease International. Available at: https://www.alzint.org/resource/world-alzheimer-report-2024/.

Alzheimer's Research UK (2023) *Dementia Attitudes Monitor: Wave 3.* Cambridge: Alzheimer's Research UK. Available at: https://www.dementiastatistics.org/attitudes/Dementia%20Attitudes%20Monitor%20-%20Wave%203%20report.pdf.

Banerjee, S. (2010) Living well with dementia – development of the national dementia strategy for England, *International Journal of Geriatric Psychiatry*, 25(9): 917–22.

Bartlett, R., Dening, T., Oliver, K., et al. (2017) Suffering with dementia: the other side of 'living well', *International Psychogeriatrics*, 29(2): 177–79.

Batchelor, A., Bingham, J., Burton, J., et al. (2023) The IDEAL Living with Dementia Toolkit: living your life with hope, *Journal of Dementia Care*, 31(1): 20–24.

Beesley, I., Hall, M., Husband, T., et al. (2020) *The Unfurlings: Banners for Hope and Change.* York: Darkroom Press.

Brookes, G. (2023) Killer, thief or companion? A corpus-based study of dementia metaphors in UK tabloids, *Metaphor and Symbol*, 38(3): 213–30.

Clare, L., Pentecost, C., Collins, R., et al. (2023) Evaluating 'living well' with mild-to-moderate dementia: co-production and validation of the IDEAL My Life Questionnaire, *Dementia*, 22(7): 1548–66.

Department of Health (2009) *Living well with dementia: A national dementia strategy.* London: Department of Health. Available at: https://www.gov.uk/government/publications/living-well-with-dementia-a-national-dementia-strategy.

Department of Health (2013) *Dementia: A state of the nation report on dementia care and support in England.* London: Department of Health. Available at: https://assets.publishing.service.gov.uk/media/5a7c5719ed915d3d0e87bba8/Dementia.pdf.

Department of Health (2015) *Prime Minister's challenge on dementia 2020.* London: Department of Health. Available at: https://www.gov.uk/government/publications/prime-ministers-challenge-on-dementia-2020.

IDEAL Programme (2021) *How are you feeling today?*, Living with Dementia Toolkit. Available at: livingwithdementiatoolkit.org.uk/home/how-are-you-feeling-today/ (accessed 10 October 2024).

IDEAL Programme (2022) *The World Turned Upside Down: Using theatre to take a realistic look at dementia.* YouTube. Available at: youtube.com/watch?v=__A255O5vAk (accessed 18 September 2024).

Kitwood, T.M. (1997) *Dementia Reconsidered: The Person Comes First.* Buckingham: Open University Press.

Mitchell, W. (2022) *What I Wish People Knew about Dementia: From Someone Who Knows*. London: Bloomsbury.

NHS England (2016) *The Well Pathway for Dementia*, NHS England. Available at: england. nhs.uk/mentalhealth/wp-content/uploads/sites/29/2016/03/dementia-well-pathway. pdf (accessed 22 September 2024).

Pentecost, C., Hunt, A., Litherland, R., et al. (2024) Qualitative evaluation of My Life Today – a co-produced personal tool from the IDEAL programme to help people with dementia monitor valued aspects of their lives, *Dementia*. Available at: https://doi. org/10.1177/14713012241306506.

Quinn, C., Pickett, J.A., Litherland, R., et al. (2022) Living well with dementia: what is possible and how to promote it, *International Journal of Geriatric Psychiatry*, 37(1): e5627. Available at: https://doi.org/10.1002/gps.5627.

Thred CIC (2022) *Brave New World*. Available at: youtube.com/watch?v=vH9dKe4-_J0 (accessed 5 September 2024).

4 Being a carer

Catherine Quinn

My greatest satisfaction is being able to carry out my daily activities and give my wife the daily help she requires. This gives me a lot of satisfaction and enables my wife to have a decent quality of life and cope better with her illness.

(A carer participating in IDEAL)

In this chapter we will:

- explore what it means to be a carer and acknowledge that carers are a diverse group with varying needs
- describe the many things that can influence carers' well-being
- understand how carers' experiences and well-being can change over time
- identify why it is important for carers to have access to appropriate support services

What is a carer?

'*I'm not a carer as such, you know, all I do is fill in the odd word that [my wife] cannot remember*' (Stapley et al., in press). The person with dementia is often, but not always, supported by someone with whom they have had a longstanding relationship. This person is often described as a family carer or an unpaid carer. This is different to a 'formal' carer, someone who is paid to provide care as part of their job. Previous chapters have explored living well in people with dementia in terms of the overall picture, diversity among different groups, and what it means for individuals. In this chapter, I focus on the family members or friends who provide support for people with dementia. Carers play a vital role in helping people with dementia to live well. This chapter will explore how they can best be supported.

Carers tend to be a person's spouse/partner, relative, or friend. How the carer is related to the person with dementia can have an influence on their experiences and expectations of the role. They may also differ in their own circumstances. For example, some may still be working, and some may not be living with the person with dementia. As we will see in the next section, it is important to consider such differences between carers and not treat all carers as the same.

Many carers do not perceive themselves to be 'carers', especially in the earlier stages of the condition, and the reasons for this can be quite complex. Providing care and support to individuals is a natural part of all relationships. The diagnosis of dementia can start to change the dynamic of a relationship, but people may not always recognise a change in roles. A person's introduction to the caring role may be very subtle. Many carers may not see themselves as 'carers'; rather, they are just helping out a family member or friend. A relationship can start to develop into more of a caring relationship when one person becomes increasingly dependent on the other for help with daily activities. With increasing dependency, caring can become the dominant part of the relationship, although this is not always the case.

Carers often start providing support even before there has been a diagnosis of dementia. However, it may only be with a formal diagnosis or the increasing support needs of the person that triggers a realisation that the carer is taking on more of a supporting role. In IDEAL, carers were asked about how they viewed their identity (Stapley et al., in press). Some did not see themselves as carers, as the term 'carer' encompassed something *'more intense, hands on. Almost a sort of physical looking after'*. Others minimised the carer 'identity', as they wanted to preserve the existing relationship. Some did see themselves more in a caring role, possibly because they were providing more hands-on care.

Given the issues around carer identity, how important is it for carers to view themselves as fulfilling that role? To some extent, it does not matter, but one area where it can be helpful to identify as a carer is in accessing support. People who see themselves as taking a caring role need to know that they can access financial, practical, or emotional support. Accessing support is crucial for both their own and the person's well-being. However, it can be harder for people to seek out and accept help if they do not perceive themselves as a carer.

Not all carers are the same

As I alluded to the start of this chapter, there are differences among carers. Keith, a member of the ALWAYs group, commented: *'Carers are unique and different and should be treated as such'*. Just as not all people with dementia are the same, not all carers are the same. They will differ in their needs and circumstances. Carers who are spouses/partners are more likely to be older, to be retired, and perceive their role as a natural continuum of their relationship. Carers who are children will be younger and may be caring on top of other responsibilities and commitments. For example, they may have families of their own who they need to support alongside the person with dementia. Carers have described the challenges of trying to balance all of these needs (Quinn et al., 2015), and may feel guilty because they do not have the time they would like to spend with these individuals. Thus, they may find themselves in the difficult position of trying to keep everyone happy.

Some carers may also have to balance caring duties with a job. In IDEAL, just over half of carers under the age of 65 were employed (Henderson et al., 2019). Trying to manage work alongside caring can be challenging. A carer may have to reduce their working hours, which will have a financial impact. In IDEAL, carers aged under 65 were more likely to have lost working hours compared to carers aged 65+ (Henderson et al., 2019). Over time, some carers reduced their working hours (Henderson et al., 2022).

Another factor to consider is the living situation of the person with dementia. In IDEAL, 285 people with dementia (18.5 per cent) lived alone (Clare et al., 2020), meaning that some carers were caring for someone they did not live with. This may be beneficial for those carers because it places a time limit on the support they can provide, as they need to go back to their own home. However, there will be some challenges. A carer may have to travel some distance to provide care, which may become tiring. With good support it is possible for some people with dementia to live independently by themselves, but carers may worry about them and feel guilty for not being available. For example, carers may feel that they cannot protect the person with dementia as they would do if they were living with them, such as checking the cooker has been switched off. Carers may also worry about the person with dementia being vulnerable and at risk of abuse. When this is the case, drawing on wider support networks can be helpful. One carer I worked with relied on a network of neighbours to 'keep an eye' on her father when she was not around.

The different types of support carers provide

Providing support to a person with dementia can be a stressful experience. It is usually not a role that someone was expecting to take on, or 'signed up for'. Carers often feel guilty that they are not doing as good a job as they ought to be doing, although as Jane, a member of the ALWAYs group, commented: *'You've got to let go of the guilt as much as you can'.*

We can divide the type of support carers provide into practical and emotional support. The amount of practical support a person with dementia needs will vary. In IDEAL, most people with dementia (87 per cent) received help from friends or relatives, usually about 36 hours per week (Henderson et al., 2019). Carers help the person with dementia with different types of activities. In IDEAL, 30 per cent of carers said they assisted with personal care, 44 per cent made sure the person was safe, 68 per cent helped with finances, 70 per cent helped with practical matters, and 74 per cent escorted the person to appointments (Henderson et al., 2019). Carers often have to take over some of the person's roles and responsibilities. They will also have to adjust to the person with dementia not being as able to support them as much. As the person's dementia progresses, it is likely the carer will have to provide more support in terms of personal care, such as shaving or bathing. Some carers feel uncomfortable having to involve themselves in these more intimate aspects of care.

Carers also provide emotional support to the person with dementia. As will be discussed in Chapter 9, the person with dementia has to deal with their diagnosis and the impact this will have on their lives. The carer may find that they are having to provide emotional support to the person as well as dealing with their own worries and concerns (Quinn et al., 2008). Part of this will involve encouraging the person to continue doing things that they are still capable of. This might be hard for carers – when they are busy or feel under pressure, it can sometimes be easier to do things themselves. However, by not letting the person with dementia do things, they are at greater risk of becoming more dependent on their carer. Monica, a member of the ALWAYs group, highlighted: *'Don't underestimate what the person with dementia can actually do or say at times'*.

The impact of caring on the carer

Providing care for someone with dementia can have a negative impact on carers. Part of this relates to the act of caring itself, but the carer will also have to adjust to the changes in the person with dementia as well as their own lives. As one carer taking part in IDEAL said:

> *I have to think for two instead of just for myself because he can't cope with any kind of stress or decision-making. That does make you feel a bit lonely sometimes because we used to talk over everything together ... at least you had a sounding board and I don't have that with him now.*

Providing care and support can be both physically and mentally exhausting and can lead to feelings of stress and burnout. On a day-to-day basis, for example, it can be tiring to deal with someone who asks what might be perceived as repetitive questions. More generally, it can be distressing to witness a decline in the person.

Some of the challenges of caring can relate to the carer's own understanding of what is happening to the person. Even with a diagnosis of dementia, the carer may struggle to link the changes they are observing to the dementia. The carer's understanding is important as it can impact on how they respond to the person with dementia. If the carer sees the behaviour as a symptom of dementia, then they are more likely to be sympathetic. However, if the carer thinks the person is purposively acting that way or 'acting-up', it is easy to become frustrated or impatient. For example, one carer I worked with got very annoyed with his wife because she kept putting the washing powder in the wrong place. In IDEAL, we looked at how carers understood dementia. Although most knew the person's diagnosis, under half used a diagnostic word, such as dementia or Alzheimer's, to refer to that person's condition (Quinn et al., 2019a). This might have been because they were trying to protect the person with dementia by not using the diagnostic word, and instead felt more comfortable referring to memory issues (Quinn et al., 2017). Carers can also struggle to understand the causes of the person's difficulties and how the condition will change over time (Quinn et al., 2019a).

The challenges associated with caring can have a negative impact on carers' well-being. In IDEAL, we found that carers experiencing higher care-related stress tended to have lower well-being and satisfaction with life (Quinn et al., 2019b). In Chapter 1, we explained how in IDEAL we looked at the overall influences on living well for people with dementia. We undertook a similar process for carers. Five of the domains were those that were applied to people with dementia. For carers, we also looked at the quality of the carer's relationship with the person with dementia and their experiences of caring. This covered areas such as care-related stress, whether anyone shared the caring role, and whether they experienced role captivity (feeling trapped in the caring role). We wished to see how these domains were linked to the carers' living well scores. Figure 4.1 shows the strength of the association between each of the domains and living well. We found that psychological characteristics and health was most strongly related to living well, followed by physical fitness and health, and experiencing caregiving. Social resources and relationship were also related, but less strongly so. Social situation and managing everyday life with dementia were not related to carers' living well scores (Clare et al., 2019).

These findings show that lots of things influence whether carers can live well, and some things may be more important than others. They highlight the importance of supporting carers' psychological and physical health. Carers need support to develop and maintain positive coping strategies. Having a strong and supportive social network, and participating in social and community activities, is also valuable. It is important that carers receive proper support to help them maintain their well-being. We used what we learned from IDEAL to develop a carers' Living with Dementia Map, shown in Figure 4.2 (explore it in full on the IDEAL website; IDEAL Programme, n.d.).

Figure 4.1: Relationship between life domains and living well for carers.

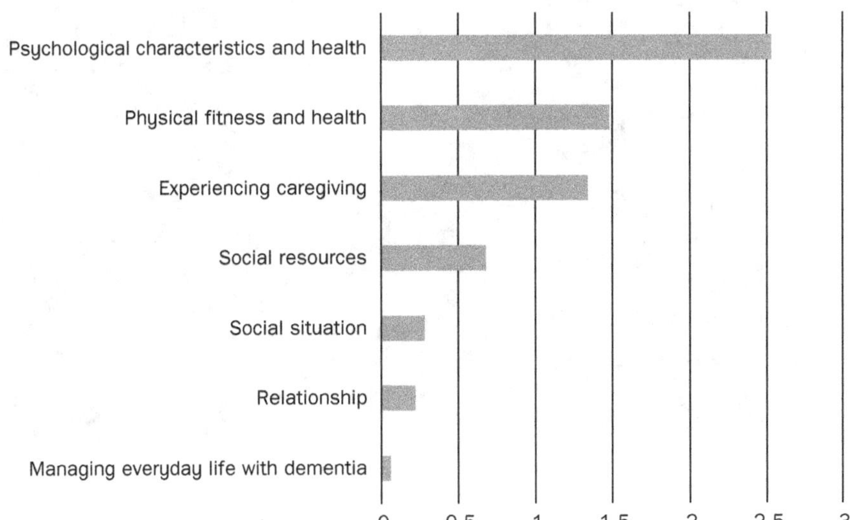

Figure 4.2: The Living with Dementia Map for carers.

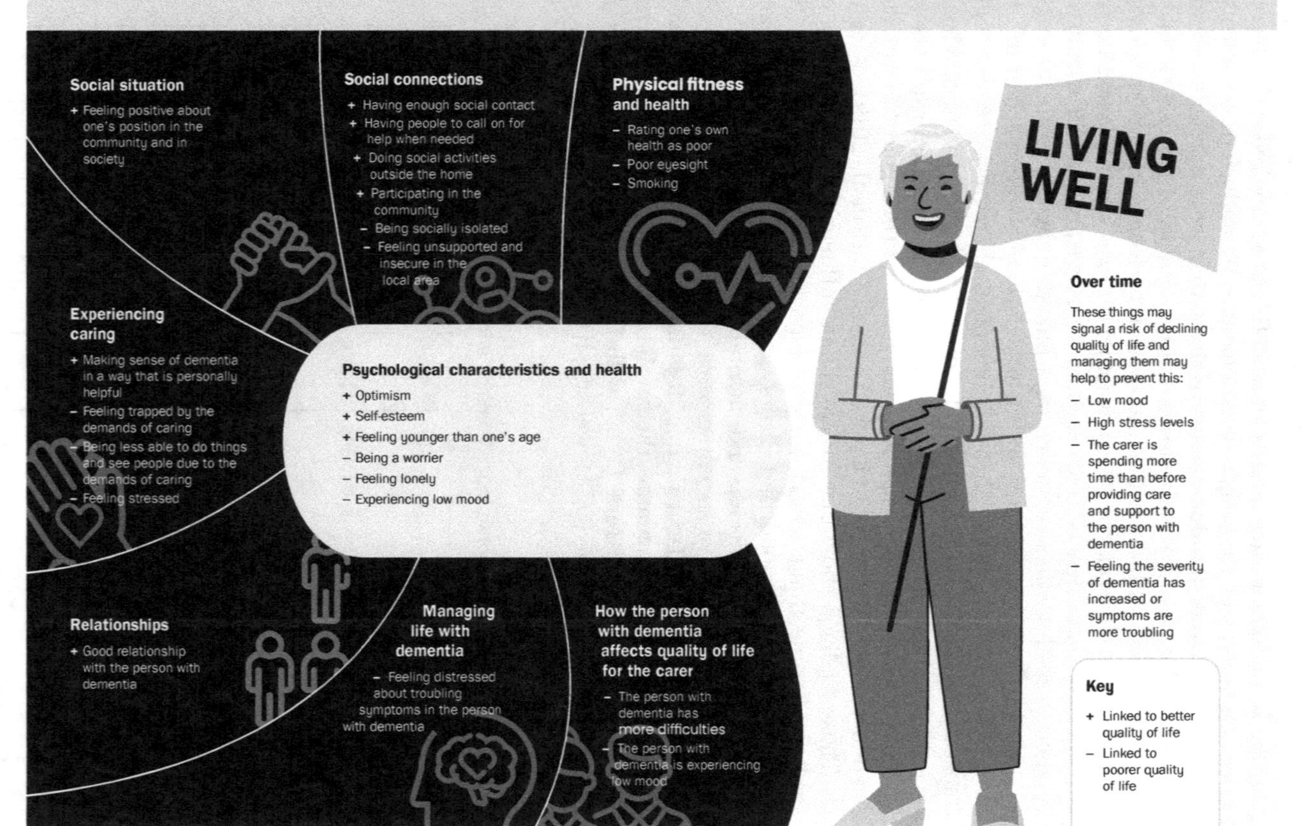

Positive experiences in providing care

So far, we have considered some of the challenges faced by carers – but some carers have positive experiences in providing care. As one of our IDEAL carers commented: '*It's doing something worthwhile that is helping the person I love*'.

When faced with challenging circumstances in life, people can experience both positive and negative emotions; these can lead them to find ways of coping with the situation. This can be likened to resilience, being able to adapt in difficult circumstances (Martyr et al., 2023). Many of the carers we spoke to in IDEAL identified having positive experiences in providing care (Quinn et al., 2024b), and this tended to continue as time progressed (Quinn et al., 2024a).

It is important to recognise, however, that the IDEAL carers were caring for people with mild-to-moderate dementia, not severe dementia. In IDEAL, carers were asked: 'What is your greatest satisfaction in caring for your relative/friend?' Of the 900 carers who responded to the question, 839 stated some sort of satisfaction; 49 could not identify any particular satisfaction and 12 were unsure. One of the main satisfactions carers identified was maintaining their relationship with the person with dementia. They talked about the importance of still being together. Some carers experienced personal growth, in that they had learned something about themselves or felt that they had developed as a person. There were opportunities to develop new skills, and seeing that they were making a difference was important to carers. They were helping the person with dementia to retain some independence and, as much as possible, live a 'normal life'.

There is some evidence that identifying with positive experiences of caring can be beneficial for the carer's well-being (Quinn et al., 2009; Quinn and Toms, 2019). In IDEAL, perceiving more positive aspects of caring was linked to better satisfaction with life and well-being (Quinn et al., 2019b). If a carer finds the role rewarding, it will also likely be beneficial for the person with dementia.

As well as caring for the person with dementia, carers need to care for themselves

It is very important for carers to look after themselves as well as the person with dementia. As Keith, a member of the ALWAYs group, said:

> *There is a reservoir of compassion and that reservoir needs re-filling; you can't keep giving and giving unless you refill and restore and replenish, otherwise you'll just go downhill yourself.*

Although carers need to look after their own needs, they may not feel they have the time to do so. In IDEAL, just over half of the carers undertook what might be considered minimal physical activity during a typical week. Many carers also have physical or mental health issues of their own to deal with while supporting the person with dementia. In IDEAL, most spousal carers had at least one health condition and almost a third had two or more health conditions (Sabatini et al., 2024). Carers may feel that they need to prioritise the needs of the person with dementia over their own needs.

It is important for carers to engage in activities that support their own well-being. In IDEAL, we found that, for spousal carers, interactions with friends and relatives were infrequent and typically less than once a month, although the carers were not socially isolated as they had friends whom they could count on (Sabatini et al., 2023). Around two-thirds of the carers in IDEAL reported feeling lonely (Victor et al., 2021b). This is higher than the level of loneliness reported among the general population of older people. Those carers who mixed with fewer people, were socially isolated, and experienced more care-related stress were more likely to report feeling lonely (Victor et al., 2021a). Allison, a member of the ALWAYs group, described how her husband's social world began to shrink upon taking on a caring role:

> *I remember when I had my diagnosis, my husband got into a stage where he felt really lonely, he felt very alone. He did not know where to go or what to do, and he felt at that stage all of his attention had to go onto me and he was cutting connections.*

In IDEAL, we also explored the impact of the COVID-19 pandemic and resulting restrictions on carers (Quinn et al., 2022a). Interestingly, during the pandemic, we found that carers had more contact with relatives than previously. They were also more likely to identify someone to share the role of carer. Despite this, however, they felt more lonely. This might have been because, although they had more contact with their relatives, it was often over the phone rather than face-to-face.

The person with dementia can also have a role in supporting the carer's well-being. Although the nature of their relationship might change, the person with dementia can still look after the carer and the importance of this should not be overlooked. By working together, the carer and person with dementia can continue to share responsibilities and concerns with one another.

Situations can change

Due to the progressive nature of dementia, there will necessarily be changes to the caring role. This could be on a day-to-day basis or over the longer term. As Jane, a member of the ALWAYs group, commented: '*Every day is not equal; what your loved one is going through, what you are going through, may change*'.

In Chapter 1, we explained how, in IDEAL, we explored whether the quality of life of people with dementia changed over time. We also looked at how things changed for carers at Times 1, 2, and 3. For most carers, well-being remained relatively stable over time. There was also a small group of carers (about 7 per cent) whose well-being declined over time (Clare et al., 2022). This seemed to be because the person with dementia developed further difficulties and needed much more support. These carers also experienced more negative emotions such as depression and role captivity (feeling trapped in the caring role). We supplemented the analyses with information from Times 4, 5, and 6 and found that there were small decreases in well-being over time. We also found that some things had 'knock-on' effects over time – for instance, having more care-related stress in one year negatively affected well-being the following year.

Looking at care-related stress in more detail, we found that for most carers, stress levels did not change much over time. Most carers had either moderate (46 per cent) or low (39.5 per cent) levels of stress, which increased slightly over time, while a minority (about 8 per cent) experienced high levels of stress which stayed the same over time. For about 6 per cent of carers, their stress levels increased quite a lot over time (Quinn et al., 2024a).

Carers also experience changes in their own role and the support needs of the person with dementia. In IDEAL, we found that over time some carers were providing more hours of care (Clare et al., 2022). The nature of their relationship with the person with dementia may also alter. They will see differences in the person, often gradual, which can be difficult to deal with as they may feel they are 'losing' that person. As a carer in IDEAL said: '*I do lose a little bit of him every month, I can see it disappearing; he doesn't remember things*'.

As carers notice more and more changes in the person, they can start to miss the role that person played in their life (Quinn et al., 2015). Carers may also start to grieve for the loss of a future together with that person, realising that things they had planned to do together are no longer feasible. Carers may have to adjust to transitional events, such as the person entering into a more formal care arrangement, and may find themselves having a diminished role in providing support for their loved one. If they shared a home with the person, they may find it difficult to adjust to living apart. Carers may also have to re-evaluate their future and begin to move on with their lives without the person with dementia.

Asking for support can be difficult

Providing support to someone with dementia can be challenging, so it is very important that carers access support services. However, as identified earlier, if someone does not perceive themselves to be a carer, they may be reluctant to seek support. It can also be difficult to contemplate involving others in the care of the person with dementia. Indeed, many carers feel they are failing in their role if they access support, as they should be able to cope by themselves.

There are also barriers to accessing support services. Societal and cultural norms may create expectations that family members will provide care (Victor et al., 2024). Carers may feel pressure from other family members to keep providing support, or feel there is no one who can help them (Quinn et al., 2015). This can make carers uncomfortable with seeking support from formal services. This can also be linked to wider issues around a lack of understanding of dementia in some communities (Victor et al., 2024). The provision of post-diagnostic support services is often patchy and ALWAYs group members describe it as a 'postcode lottery', which means the support you can access will vary depending on where you live. Carers may not be aware of what support is available to them, and it can be difficult to know where to start when seeking support (Quinn et al., 2022b). In IDEAL, both carers and people with dementia identified the need for better signposting to services (Quinn et al., 2022b). Carers identified that services need to be designed to deliver support in a more culturally inclusive way. In the Living with Dementia Toolkit (IDEAL Programme, 2021), introduced in Chapter 3, the 'Stay Positive' section highlights the value of carers meeting with other carers. Although it can be tricky for carers to find appropriate services, as shown in the banner developed by Oldham Dementia Carers in Figure 4.3, there are different types of support out there.

Figure 4.3: Oldham Dementia Carers banner 'We are here and We care'.

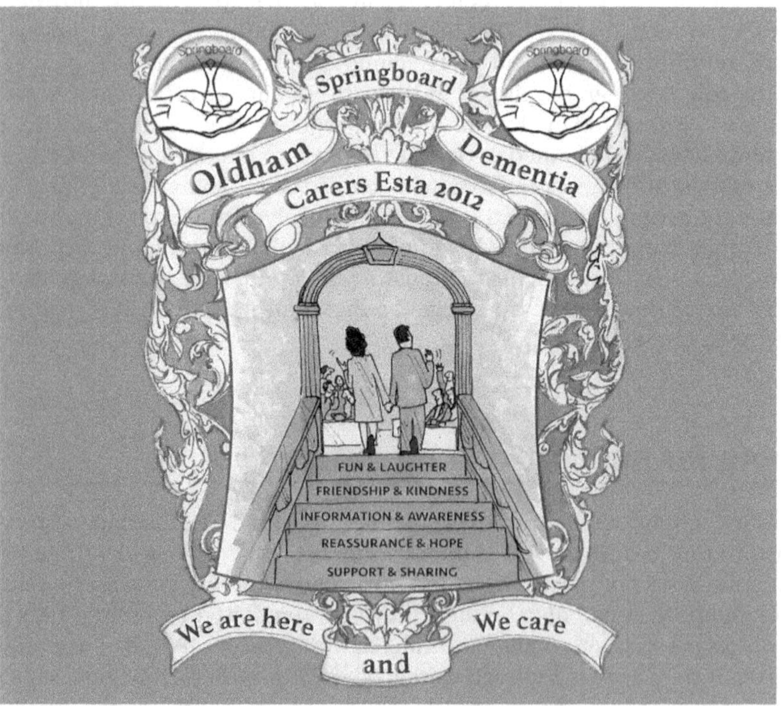

So what does this tell us about reconsidering living with dementia?

As part of IDEAL, we have shown that we need to rethink how we understand carers. Carers are not all the same and should not be treated as such. It is often thought that the support carers provide is 'free', yet providing support comes at a considerable cost to carers' well-being and other aspects of their lives, such as having to cut back on working hours. We have to rethink our understanding of the things that influence carers' well-being. This includes looking beyond care-related stress and recognising that other things, such as carers' psychological health and physical health, have an impact on their well-being. We also need to acknowledge that some carers have positive experiences. It is important that we explore all these different aspects when assessing carers' needs. In IDEAL, we found that many carers' well-being declined over time. Support services need to be better at spotting those at risk.

These findings show that we need to rethink the support that is available to carers. Support is often focused on the period immediately after diagnosis and as our ALWAYs group identified, this is a 'postcode lottery'. Yet this chapter has highlighted that support needs change over time, and it is vital that support services are responsive to this. We also have to recognise that not all carers will identify as 'carers'; we need ways of identifying these individuals and making them feel it is perfectly okay for them to accept help. Ultimately, to enable carers to live well, they need access to appropriate support services, which they should be directed to rather than seek out themselves. This should lead to more effective and individualised support provision. As one of the carers we spoke to in IDEAL said: '*[You need] somebody who cares about how you're coping. Not a lot to ask*'.

Reflections from the ALWAYs group

We reflected on the challenges of the caring role, noting that every day is different, and the situation can be unpredictable. We recognised that for some, the need to care for a person with dementia is a daunting and unwanted experience. We recognised that carers may feel guilty or feel judged for not being able to fulfill the role in a way that they would have wished. We also found that the findings from IDEAL, which show that there are positive qualities about the life of a carer, were uplifting and helpful.

We realise that knowledge and understanding of caring is often acquired through hindsight. This highlights gaps in the support provided to carers. On reflecting on the contents of this chapter, we wanted to emphasise the importance of health and social care professionals being more proactive in monitoring carers. This could be through checking in with carers to see how they are coping and reminding carers of the support available as time goes by. This type of approach needs to become standard practice, rather than only in times of crisis.

> **Key points**
>
> **Key points for people with dementia and carers**
>
> - If you are a carer, it is important that you make time to look after yourself as well as the person with dementia.
> - Do not feel guilty about asking for help.
> - Try to maintain your own activities and interests; some of these can be shared together and others done independently.
>
> **Key points for health and social care practitioners**
>
> - As well as speaking to carers about the stresses of providing care, ask them about positive experiences.
> - Carers need access to holistic support that is tailored to their needs.
> - Carers' needs will change over time, so they need to be able to access support on a continuous basis.
>
> **Key points for policy-makers**
>
> - Carers are not all the same and policies should acknowledge their differing needs.
> - Recognise that support services for carers are vital and require proper investment.
> - Carers need access to dedicated support services that offer them support throughout the caring journey.

> **⚑ Manifesto statement**
>
> The well-being of the carer is as important as that of the person living with dementia: we want both to be supported.

References

Clare, L., Wu, Y.-T., Quinn, C., et al. (2019) A comprehensive model of factors associated with capability to 'live well' for family caregivers of people living with mild-to-moderate dementia: findings from the IDEAL study, *Alzheimer Disease and Associated Disorders*, 33(1): 29–35.

Clare, L., Martyr, A., Henderson, C., et al. (2020) Living alone with mild-to-moderate dementia: findings from the IDEAL cohort, *Journal of Alzheimer's Disease*, 78(3): 1207–16.

Clare, L., Gamble, L.D., Martyr, A., et al. (2022) 'Living Well' trajectories among family caregivers of people with mild-to-moderate dementia in the IDEAL cohort, *Journals of Gerontology B: Psychological Sciences and Social Sciences*, 77(10): 1852–63.

Henderson, C., Knapp, M., Nelis, S.M., et al. (2019) Use and costs of services and unpaid care for people with mild-to-moderate dementia: baseline results from the IDEAL cohort study, *Alzheimer's and Dementia: Translational Research and Clinical Interventions*, 5(1): 685–96.

Henderson, C., Knapp, M., Martyr, A., et al. (2022) The use and costs of paid and unpaid care for people with dementia: longitudinal findings from the IDEAL cohort, *Journal of Alzheimer's Disease*, 86(1): 135–53.

IDEAL Programme (2021) *Sharing is caring*, Living with Dementia Toolkit. Available at: livingwithdementiatoolkit.org.uk/stay-positive/sharing-is-caring/ (accessed 7 August 2024).

IDEAL Programme (n.d.) *Living with dementia maps*. Available at: www.idealproject. org.uk/projects/maps (accessed 14 September 2024).

Martyr, A., Rusted, J.M., Quinn, C., et al. (2023) Resilience in caregivers of people with mild-to-moderate dementia: findings from the IDEAL cohort, *BMC Geriatrics*, 23(1): 804. Available at: https://doi.org/10.1186/s12877-023-04549-y.

Quinn, C. and Toms, G. (2019) Influence of positive aspects of dementia caregiving on caregivers' well-being: a systematic review, *The Gerontologist*, 59(5): e584–96. Available at: https://doi.org/10.1093/geront/gny168.

Quinn, C., Clare, L. and Woods, R.T. (2009) The impact of motivations and meanings on the wellbeing of caregivers of people with dementia: a systematic review, *International Psychogeriatrics*, 22(1): 43–55.

Quinn, C., Clare, L. and Woods, R.T. (2015) Balancing needs: the role of motivations, meanings and relationship dynamics in the experience of informal caregivers of people with dementia, *Dementia*, 14(2): 220–37.

Quinn, C., Jones, I.R. and Clare, L. (2017) Illness representations in caregivers of people with dementia, *Aging and Mental Health*, 21(5): 553–61.

Quinn, C., Clare, L., Pearce, A., et al. (2008) The experience of providing care in the early stages of dementia: an interpretative phenomenological analysis, *Aging and Mental Health*, 12(6): 769–78.

Quinn, C., Jones, I.R., Martyr, A., et al. (2019a) Caregivers' beliefs about dementia: findings from the IDEAL study, *Psychology and Health*, 34(10): 1214–30.

Quinn, C., Nelis, S.M., Martyr, A., et al. (2019b) Influence of positive and negative dimensions of dementia caregiving on caregiver well-being and satisfaction with life: findings from the IDEAL study, *American Journal of Geriatric Psychiatry*, 27(8): 838–48.

Quinn, C., Gamble, L.D., Parker, S., et al. (2022a) Impact of COVID-19 on carers of people with dementia in the community: findings from the British IDEAL cohort, *International Journal of Geriatric Psychiatry*, 37(5): e5708. Available at: https://doi. org/10.1002/gps.5708.

Quinn, C., Hart, N., Henderson, C., et al. (2022b) Developing supportive local communities: perspectives from people with dementia and caregivers participating in the IDEAL programme, *Journal of Aging and Social Policy*, 34(6): 1–21.

Quinn, C., Gamble, L.D., Morris, R.G., et al. (2024a) Longitudinal trajectories of stress and positive aspects of dementia caregiving: findings from the IDEAL programme, *Journals of Gerontology B: Psychological Sciences and Social Sciences*, 79(8): gbae097. Available at: https://doi.org/10.1093/geronb/gbae097.

Quinn, C., Toms, G., Rippon, I., et al. (2024b) Positive experiences in dementia caregiving: findings from the IDEAL programme, *Ageing and Society*, 44(5): 1010–30.

Sabatini, S., Martyr, A., Gamble, L.D., et al. (2023) Profiles of social, cultural, and economic capital as longitudinal predictors of stress, positive experiences of caring, and depression among carers of people with dementia, *Aging and Mental Health*, 27(7): 1335–43.

Sabatini, S., Martyr, A., Hunt, A., et al. (2024) Health conditions in spousal caregivers of people with dementia and their relationships with stress, caregiving experiences, and social networks: longitudinal findings from the IDEAL programme, *BMC Geriatrics*, 24(1): 171. Available at: https://doi.org/10.1186/s12877-024-04707-w.

Stapley, S., Pentecost, C., Hillman, A., et al. (submitted) Negotiating the caring role and carer identity over time: 'living well' and the longitudinal narratives of family members of people with dementia from the IDEAL cohort, *Ageing & Society*. Available at: https://doi.org/10.1017/S0144686X25000030.

Victor, C.R., Rippon, I., Quinn, C., et al. (2021a) The role of subjective social status in living well for carers of people with dementia: findings from the Improving the experience of Dementia and Enhancing Active Life programme, *International Journal of Care and Caring*, 5(3): 447–67.

Victor, C.R., Rippon, I., Quinn, C., et al. (2021b) The prevalence and predictors of loneliness in caregivers of people with dementia: findings from the IDEAL programme, *Aging and Mental Health*, 25(7): 1232–38.

Victor, C.R., van den Heuvel, E., Pentecost, C., et al. (2024) Perspectives of minority ethnic caregivers of people with dementia interviewed as part of the IDEAL programme, *Health and Social Care in the Community*, 2024: 8732644. Available at: https://doi.org/10.1155/2024/8732644.

5 Feeling part of the world: social connections

Claire Pentecost and Christina Victor

> *This business of living well, it is a lonely existence unless I/we make an effort to communicate with others.*
>
> (Person with dementia; Quinn et al., 2022b: 848)
>
> *It's good to be able to do something that keeps you occupied … And feel that you're part of the world.*
>
> (Person with dementia; Stapley et al., 2023: 13)

In this chapter we will:

- consider why being socially connected is so important to the well-being of people with dementia
- understand how where we live influences well-being, and consider the challenges faced by people with dementia who live alone or who feel lonely
- highlight what we can do to support people with dementia to express their views and to be socially engaged
- focus on the need for people, communities, and society to be inclusive

What is social connection and why is it important?

Human beings are social creatures, and there is strong evidence that being connected is beneficial to our health and well-being. Social connectedness is a feeling of belonging to a group and generally feeling close to other people. It has been defined as 'the degree to which people have and perceive a desired number, quality, and diversity of relationships that create a sense of belonging, and being cared for, valued and supported' (US Centers for Disease Control and Prevention, 2024).

The challenges of loneliness and isolation

Social connections are good for our mental and physical well-being, and the opposite is true for those feeling lonely or isolated. A person who feels lonely experiences a disconnection between their desire for a certain quantity and quality of relationships and what is available to them (Perlman and Peplau, 1981), while a socially isolated person has a small social network that they engage with infrequently. Both loneliness and isolation are bad for the well-being of individuals and several countries have dedicated loneliness strategies, with campaigns run by third-sector organisations to tackle the problem.

In IDEAL, we wanted to see whether people with dementia were lonelier or more isolated than other older people because these two factors are an important influence on the ability to live well for people with dementia. Levels of loneliness among people with dementia who took part in IDEAL were high. Roughly one in three (35 per cent) experienced moderate or severe loneliness and 15 per cent were socially isolated: levels comparable with the general population of older people (Victor et al., 2020).

We did not find any differences in loneliness or isolation between people with dementia who lived in urban or rural areas or who lived in deprived or more advantaged areas, or who did or did not have access to nature in nearby blue or green spaces. One group at higher risk of experiencing loneliness or isolation was those who lived alone. In the IDEAL study, almost a fifth of people with dementia lived alone (Clare et al., 2020). This group were older and more likely to be female, had fewer difficulties with memory, and were also better able to manage the everyday activities needed to remain independent than those living with others. However, they were more likely to feel lonely and had higher levels of isolation than those who lived with others.

Work by Dementia Enquirers in the UK shows that some people with dementia feel living alone has some advantages, such as fewer arguments, fewer difficulties from poor relationships, and less need to depend on others (Dementia Enquirers, 2021). People living alone made efforts to be involved in meetings and connect with a range of people, although loneliness could be an issue in the evenings. This illustrates the point that many people with dementia living alone find ways to maintain heathy social relationships. However, those who have few social contacts or are known to be lonely may also have little social support. Providing opportunities for social interaction where it is missing, or care and support at times when loneliness is heightened, may help to promote good social health.

Personal connection

Central to social connection is the ability to communicate ideas, wishes, views, and experiences to others. People with dementia have told us that they are not always asked, heard, or understood. The value of spending time with people was succinctly described by a man with dementia we interviewed during the pandemic: '*That emotion you feel from a visit far outstrips any good news that might have been imparted because you won't remember that. But it's the emotional feeling that ... you are left with*' (Stapley et al., 2023: 14).

It is important to include people with dementia in conversations that may affect their lives and enable them to contribute to wider society. Speaking with people with dementia during IDEAL revealed key areas where people told us they need to be heard. These include interactions with family and friends, the wider public, and health professionals, especially when dementia becomes more severe.

Personal interactions with family and friends

We have heard about things that can be difficult to broach in families during the IDEAL research. This came to the fore when developing scenes for the IDEAL play 'The World Turned Upside Down' (IDEAL Programme, 2022a). The effect of noticing a decline in the person with dementia was depicted in a scene involving a conversation between a father and daughter about whether he was still safe to drive a car, as shown in the photograph below.

Scene from The World Turned Upside Down: is it safe to drive?

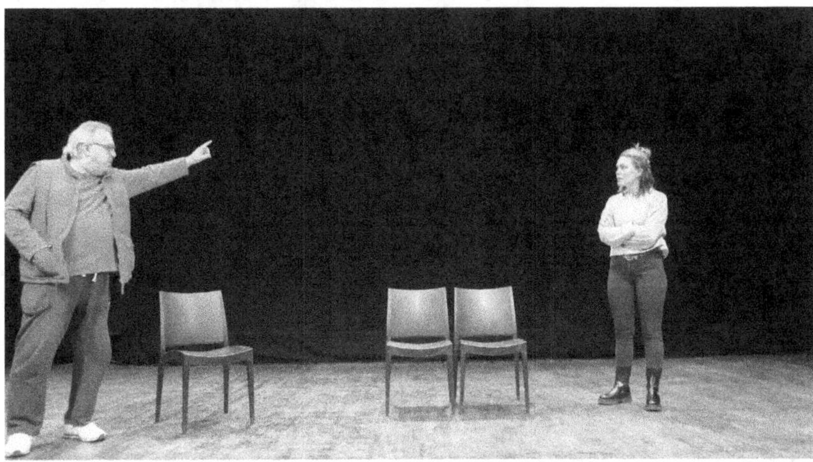

The scene highlighted how the dynamics of the relationship between a parent and adult child could make that already-difficult conversation even harder. When communicating with people who are close to us, we may be naturally more cautious to avoid damaging the relationship. Sensitivity and selflessness, alongside a willingness to listen, can enable both individuals to truly understand each other and to reach a compromise. These delicate conversations are far from easy, and in thinking about planning for the future, it is useful to talk about things as early as possible, well before reaching a crisis point. This means decisions can be negotiated and made jointly.

Meeting other people with dementia

Connections with other people with dementia can offer peer support – the opportunity to learn about the experiences of other people who have dementia. This sort of support is especially valuable as it gives the chance to interact with people who really understand. It helps people to realise they are not alone, and they learn from the positive stories and practical tips other people have learned along the way. People with dementia benefit from their involvement with dementia-specific groups or peer support groups where they can relax because they are with other '*people who get it*' (Person with dementia; Dawson et al., 2023: 775). There is information about peer support in the 'Stay connected' section of the Living with Dementia Toolkit (IDEAL Programme, 2022b).

Local community groups for people with dementia such as memory cafés and meeting centres have been developing rapidly internationally to help reduce loneliness and isolation for people with dementia and their families. They are places people with dementia can go for practical information, personal advice, and emotional and social support from trained staff and volunteers, and from the other people with dementia attending. There is good evidence to show that attending can have positive benefits on self-esteem, emotions, and feelings of belonging (Brooker et al., 2018).

There are also opportunities to meet and develop friendships online and there are groups in many countries, such as those offered by the Alzheimer's Association in the US (Alzheimer's Association, 2024) and DEEP, the UK network of dementia voices (DEEP, 2024). The latter offers a good example of how to support engagement by helping people get online and use apps like Zoom (Dementia Voices, 2019). Information about online or face-to-face resources can be found by searching online or asking local dementia organisations.

Meeting the needs of people with changes in speech or language

Barriers to effective communication are more evident for people with dementia who experience changes to their speech and language capabilities. Some dementias such as certain variants of frontotemporal dementia are characterised by aphasia (difficulties with understanding, speaking, reading, or writing) from an early stage. Similar difficulties can develop in other types of dementia as these progress. When these difficulties become apparent, often assumptions are made that people with dementia lack the ability to communicate meaningfully, as one dementia researcher pointed out:

> People are unaware of communicative capabilities of people with advanced dementia. In people with autism or young infants, if they are engaging in repetitive behaviours, they are always credited with some meaning, but in advanced dementia they are not. They are often thought of as meaningless, random or problematic.
>
> (Collins et al., 2022: 1141)

We wanted to explore ways of communicating that could help to challenge these assumptions and encourage inclusion of the perspectives of people with more advanced dementia. We talked to practitioners and researchers who were experienced in communicating with people living with severe dementia (Collins et al., 2022). They emphasised the importance of knowing the person, being flexible, and thinking creatively about interactions. Communication should be as straightforward as possible, for example using short sentences, avoiding direct questions, and being alert to non-verbal signs.

Any communication requires humanity and compassion to be able to observe and respond, and to adapt and change the approach to suit the individual. We have also learned from talking to people with dementia and carers about appropriate communication techniques, and information is available in the 'Stay connected' section of the Living with Dementia Toolkit (IDEAL Programme, 2022c). In a conversation with the ALWAYs group, Julia gave an example of meeting a relative with dementia at a family event:

> *I did not rush up and throw my arms around her, other people did, I saw that later and she just did not like it, especially when a little boy who was her grandson comes dressed up as Batman or something in a little mask, you know, all those difficult things. And she did not want to be ... so I sat there and waited till she saw me. And eventually it got through, something got through and it's like a waking up. In the context, the connection must be made slowly. I think a hug works, but it is not the first thing that you do.*
>
> (Julia, ALWAYs group member)

Everyone needs to take the responsibility for ensuring that people with more severe dementia are not ignored, but rather included and encouraged to express their views. This may mean adjusting how we normally communicate. Unfortunately, this does not always happen, as demonstrated in the IDEAL opera 'The Bridge'. When the person with dementia is ignored in favour of asking his wife about his preferences, he responds: '*We are in here. Look at me and communicate even if I don't answer back*' (IDEAL Programme, 2023).

Feeling included in your community can make a difference

As well as personal interactions, another aspect of social connection is engagement with wider society. People with dementia simply want to be able to live their lives in ways that allow them to continue to interact within their community and take part in activities such as voting in elections, using public facilities like libraries or parks, or supporting voluntary groups. While strong social ties to family and friends are important, the value of micro-connections that occur during these activities was mentioned during discussions with people with dementia and may be especially valued by people with fewer social connections, or those who are lonely. This is illustrated by a man with dementia who spoke of going out for a walk every day during COVID-19 restrictions to remain socially engaged: *'I've met some very nice people, and we were able to sort of have a brief talk and jokes and things like that, but still keeping our two metres apart, that sort of thing'* (Pentecost et al., 2022: 5).

We learned from the pandemic that chance meetings with people are important opportunities for connection, but our ALWAYs group have pointed out that opportunities in society to have 'micro connections' with people have become fewer in recent years. Medical appointments can be virtual instead of face-to-face, we are encouraged to use self-service checkouts at the supermarket, and a ticket machine is the only way to purchase a train ticket in many stations. Problems with how people with dementia are treated in the general community is another issue that has been raised by IDEAL research. We asked people with dementia 'What do you think could be changed in the local community to enable people like yourself to live well?'; they said they wanted better understanding of dementia within local communities, access to support and healthcare services, access to activities and outdoor environments, and opportunities to socialise and get involved. Common to all of these, and important for both people with dementia and carers, was the need for everyone in society to have a better understanding of the difficulties dementia creates in doing the things that most people do without thinking. Feeling more understood for people with dementia meant being treated as a person, which results in reduced feelings of shame, and increased awareness in shops and services so allowances can be made, for example, with things like getting muddled with money (Quinn et al., 2022b).

Concerns about how other people will respond and their lack of understanding create a feeling of an unsympathetic environment, and the associated stigma makes it more difficult for people with dementia to engage: *'You talk less because you don't want to be highlighting it [difficulties communicating]. And that, then, is like a vicious downward spiral, isn't it?'* (Dawson et al., 2023: 773). Another person with dementia commented: *'Alzheimer's is a silent menace and there is no way for people to be aware of it like people with blindness have a white stick. The only way you can let them know is by saying, and sometimes people don't want to do this'* (Quinn et al., 2022b: 10).

Campaigns and services to improve social engagement

There is international recognition of the additional challenges faced by older people in remaining socially engaged, and several national campaigns have set out to address this (World Health Organization, 2021). Although successes have been identified by encouraging groups and organisations to follow guidelines and demonstrate they are 'dementia-friendly', only half of the carers surveyed in IDEAL thought they were living in a dementia-friendly community (DFC; Quinn et al., 2022a). Our carer participants have indicated an ongoing need for training for people in public-facing organisations and services to have a better awareness of dementia, and for better layout of the physical environment to make places like supermarkets less confusing. Also, importantly, relatively few DFC initiatives have evaluated their impact and so evidence on which to base future planning is badly needed (Buckner et al., 2019). Future support for such schemes is not assured.

Difficulties accessing social activities

Meaningful engagement in social activities can give us a sense of purpose and reinforce our sense of personal identity. However, people taking part in IDEAL generally had very low levels of social participation. Participation in cultural activities averaged less than once a year for most people, which was surprising considering the people we studied lived in the community, had mild-to-moderate dementia, and had a broad age range between 43 and 98 years (Sabatini et al., 2023). People living in areas with poorer transport links and less provision of social and cultural events will be at a disadvantage and some people may prefer non-social activities. Aside from possible provision and access difficulties, not everyone feels confident mixing with other people, which can lead to a downward spiral of increasing isolation: '*You avoid people more and more, and the level of isolation gets bigger and bigger*' (person with dementia; Dawson et al., 2023: 773).

For people who prefer not to participate in organised activities or find this difficult, there are other options for remaining in contact with someone, such as befriending services. These schemes are popular worldwide and are usually designed to be friendly rather than to offer support or advice. Their usefulness was highlighted in IDEAL interviews with people with dementia during the COVID-19 pandemic when people wanted to continue with calls even when normal socialising returned (Pentecost et al., 2022).

People will have different motivations for wanting to be socially connected and will have different concerns and abilities or awareness of what is on offer locally. Personal preferences and opportunities for choice and autonomy should be valued in any service provision or when offering information to people with dementia, alongside removing as many social and local access barriers as possible. A better understanding of local needs can allow for appropriate planning and funding to support people with dementia and help them to feel more included. For example, many of us enjoy engaging with the natural world. It is beneficial for health and can be a way of connecting with like-minded people. For people with dementia who want to get out into nature, it can be hard. Places and facilities may not be accessible, transport may not be available, and cost can be an issue (Collins et al., 2023). We asked people in the IDEAL study whether they had green spaces such as parks or gardens, or blue spaces such as lakes or rivers, within a 10 minute walk of their home. The people who said they did also rated their quality of life more positively than those who said they did not. This was especially so if they lived in an urban area rather than in the countryside (Wu et al., 2021). The difference was not about whether green or blue spaces were present, but whether people were aware of them. We thought that being aware of these spaces meant that people were likely to value them and to be visiting and using them. One possible route to supporting individual preferences is by thinking about the activities that may appeal to different people with dementia and how to make them more accessible. It led us to set up a new project working with organisations that provide access to outdoor spaces to make what they offer more dementia-accessible (Stapley et al., 2024). The findings are likely to have implications for the provision of other types of activities that people with dementia may wish to participate in. Exploring personal preferences for engagement and how they can be met in people's local communities in this way lies at the heart of personalised care and support.

So what does this tell us about reconsidering living with dementia?

Engaging with our local community and wider society is an important aspect of maintaining our social networks and avoiding isolation. What we have learned from our IDEAL participants is that while most people with dementia are engaged with their family and friends, there is often limited engagement with the wider community. For both people with dementia and their carers, trust in neighbours and feeling valued by the community and wider society were linked with quality of life, well-being, and satisfaction with life. These findings emphasise the importance of building dementia-friendly communities and similar initiatives to promote a more positive approach to those with dementia or with caring responsibilities and enhance their overall ability to live well.

Reflections from the ALWAYs group

We are very aware of the importance of social connections for people with dementia and how meaningful it is to be treated with understanding, kindness, and compassion in the community even if the interactions are short.

We also recognise that some people enjoy solitude and can be happy in their own company, but where company is lacking or missed there can be a problem. We wanted to highlight that practitioners should be aware of the risk of loneliness not just for people with dementia, but also for carers, and should acknowledge and attempt to assist with the potential adverse effect on well-being.

We realise that maintaining existing friendships and connections can take work, and we should also be open to making new ones. If you are on your own, connecting with yourself in the things you do is also very important, as is getting involved with things to feel connected to others.

We understand that carers may be reluctant to take someone to a group as they may have low expectations of the possible benefit or concerns about seeing people whose dementia is more advanced and can be less willing to try new things.

We have noticed that physical touch can be a great way to communicate with a person with more advanced dementia, but it should not be the first approach; caution should be taken not to surprise them or to assume it is wanted. We should also assume in the first instance that the person can understand and wants to contribute their view, and find ways of understanding them, rather than not try.

Key points

Key points for people with dementia and carers

- Good interactions with people and groups are useful for your health and well-being.
- Find ways to keep interacting with people that you are comfortable with and let other people know if you need help. Sources of information for local activities and groups include the library, your GP, and others in your community.
- It can be useful to share your views and experiences with others; you are not alone.
- Some issues can be embarrassing or scary to talk about, but it is important to have these conversations at an early stage, so these issues do not become exacerbated in the future.

Key points for health and social care practitioners

- Understand the implications of loneliness for both people with dementia and carers.
- Identify people who are lonely, or may be at greater risk of being lonely, as they may have additional needs that can be addressed.

- People with dementia may need additional support to stay involved, engaged and sociable, and so mapping out local provision for people to connect with each other and signposting to local dementia and other community groups and services may be helpful.
- Take time and make special efforts to understand what is important to people with dementia – they may be struggling to communicate their view.
- Understand local and personal barriers to getting out and involved and help identify suitable opportunities to engage with others.

Key points for policy-makers

- Campaigns to increase public awareness of dementia that support the inclusion of people with dementia in society can make a difference.
- Peer support groups are a vital and relatively low-cost resource that should be available in all communities.
- Involve local people with dementia in the planning and implementation of local services, groups, and events.

Manifesto statement

We want to be included as active members of our communities and wider society, with opportunities to grow and maintain meaningful social connections.

References

Alzheimer's Association (2024) *ALZConnected*. Available at: alzconnected.org/ (accessed 30 July 2024).

Brooker, D., Evans, S., Evans, S., et al. (2018) Evaluation of the implementation of Meeting Centres Support Programme: the impact on people living with dementia in Italy, Poland and UK; exploration of the effects on people with dementia, *International Journal of Geriatric Psychiatry*, 33(7): 883–92.

Buckner, S., Darlington, N., Woodward, M., et al. (2019) Dementia friendly communities in England: a scoping study, *International Journal of Geriatric Psychiatry*, 34(8): 1235-1243.

Clare, L., Martyr, A., Henderson, C., et al. (2020) Living alone with mild-to-moderate dementia: findings from the IDEAL cohort, *Journal of Alzheimer's Disease*, 78(3): 1207–16.

Collins, R., Hunt, A., Quinn, C., et al. (2022) Methods and approaches for enhancing communication with people with moderate-to-severe dementia that can facilitate their inclusion in research and service evaluation: findings from the IDEAL programme, *Dementia*, 21(4): 1135–53.

Collins, R., Owen, S., Opdebeeck, C., et al. (2023) Provision of outdoor nature-based activity for older people with cognitive impairment: a scoping review from the

ENLIVEN Project, *Health and Social Care in the Community*, 2023: 4574072. Available at: https://doi.org/10.1155/2023/4574072.

Dawson, E., Collins, R., Pentecost, C., et al. (2023) Navigating the coronavirus pandemic 2 years on: experiences of people with dementia from the British IDEAL cohort, *Dementia*, 22(4): 760–82.

DEEP (2024) *Find a DEEP group in your region.* Available at: www.dementiavoices. org.uk/deep-groups/find-a-deep-group-in-your-region/ (accessed 29 July 2024).

Dementia Enquirers (2021) *The pros, cons and particular needs of those living alone with dementia and those living with a care partner.* Available at: dementiaenquirers. org.uk/projects/minds-voices-york/ (accessed 29 July 2024).

Dementia Voices (2019) *Zoomettes guide to Zoom.* Available at: www.dementiavoices. org.uk/wp-content/uploads/2019/10/Zoomettes-Guide-to-ZOOM-Version-Dec-2019.pdf (accessed 29 July 2024).

IDEAL Programme (2022a) *The World Turned Upside Down.* Available at: www.youtube. com/watch?v=__A255O5vAk&t=1s (accessed 29 July 2024).

IDEAL Programme (2022b) *Stay connected/meet other people with dementia*, Living with Dementia Toolkit. Available at: livingwithdementiatoolkit.org.uk/stay-connected/ meet-other-people-with-dementia/ (accessed 29 July 2024).

IDEAL Programme (2022c) *Stay connected*, Living with Dementia Toolkit. Available at: livingwithdementiatoolkit.org.uk/stay-connected/ (accessed 29 July 2024).

IDEAL Programme (2023) *The Bridge.* Available at: www.youtube.com/watch?v=u1t-fmA13rBYth (accessed 29 July 2024).

Pentecost, C., Collins, R., Stapley, S., et al. (2022) Effects of social restrictions on people with dementia and carers during the pre-vaccine phase of the COVID-19 pandemic: experiences of IDEAL cohort participants, *Health and Social Care in the Community*, 30(6): e4594–604. Available at: https://doi.org/10.1111/hsc.13863.

Perlman, D. and Peplau, L. (1981) Toward a social psychology of loneliness, in D.R. Gilmour (ed.) *Personal Relationships 3: Personal Relationships in Disorder.* London: Academic Press.

Quinn, C., Gamble, L.D., Parker, S., et al. (2022a) Impact of COVID-19 on carers of people with dementia in the community: findings from the British IDEAL cohort, *International Journal of Geriatric Psychiatry*, 37(5): 1–11.

Quinn, C., Hart, N., Henderson, C., et al. (2022b) Developing supportive local communities: perspectives from people with dementia and caregivers participating in the IDEAL programme, *Journal of Aging and Social Policy*, 34(6): 839–59.

Sabatini, S., Martyr, A., Gamble, L.D., et al. (2023) Are profiles of social, cultural, and economic capital related to living well with dementia? Longitudinal findings from the IDEAL programme, *Social Science and Medicine*, 317: 115603. Available at: https:// doi.org/10.1016/j.socscimed.2022.115603.

Stapley, S., Pentecost, C., Collins, R., et al. (2023) Living with dementia during the COVID-19 pandemic: insights into identity from the IDEAL cohort, *Ageing and Society.* Available at: https://doi.org/10.1017/S0144686X22001350.

Stapley, S., Wheat, H., Owen, S., et al. (2024) The dementia-nature-inclusivity nexus and the needs of people affected by dementia, *Ageing and Society.* Available at: https:// doi.org/10.1017/S0144686X24000199.

US Centers for Disease Control and Prevention (2024) *How does social connectedness affect health?* Available at: www.cdc.gov/emotional-wellbeing/social-connectedness/ affect-health.htm (accessed 29 July 2024).

Victor, C.R., Rippon, I., Nelis, S.M., et al. (2020) Prevalence and determinants of loneliness in people living with dementia: findings from the IDEAL programme, *International Journal of Geriatric Psychiatry*, 35(8): 851–58.

World Health Organization (WHO) (2021) *Towards a dementia-inclusive society: WHO toolkit for dementia-friendly initiatives (DFIs)*. Available at: www.who.int/publications/i/item/9789240031531 (accessed 29 July 2024).

Wu, Y.-T., Clare, L., Jones, I.R., et al. (2021) Perceived and objective availability of green and blue spaces and quality of life in people with dementia: results from the IDEAL programme, *Social Psychiatry and Psychiatric Epidemiology*, 56(9): 1601–10.

6 We're in this together: relationships

Catherine Quinn

I made a vow when I married him for better or for worse, in sickness and in health. We have had our good health and now we have sickness. We love each other so we work together to get through it.

(A carer participating in IDEAL)

In this chapter we will:

- explore why and how dementia can affect the relationship between the person with dementia and carer
- explore how the quality of this relationship can have an impact on the well-being of the person with dementia and carer
- explore how dementia can lead to transitions within the relationship

Different types of supportive relationship

This chapter focuses on the relationship between the person with dementia and their carer. We can consider these individuals as forming a couple or what we will refer to in this chapter as a 'dyad'. Of course, some people will have more than one carer, and there are cases where a child cares for both parents. Dementia often occurs within the context of longstanding relationships. That was the experience of Jane, a member of the ALWAYs group, who cared for her mother Ella; the photograph on the following page shows them at home together. These relationships could be spousal/partner relationships, parent-child relationships, or friendships, and it is these types of relationships this chapter will draw on. The type of relationship can have an impact on people's expectations of the relationship. For instance, spouses/partners may have more of an expectation that they will need to provide support to their spouse/partner. Children may experience more of a change in the balance of their relationship as, instead of their parent looking after them, they find they are having to provide more support to their parent. How people adjust to changes in the relationship due to dementia will often relate to these pre-existing relationships.

Jane and her mother Ella.

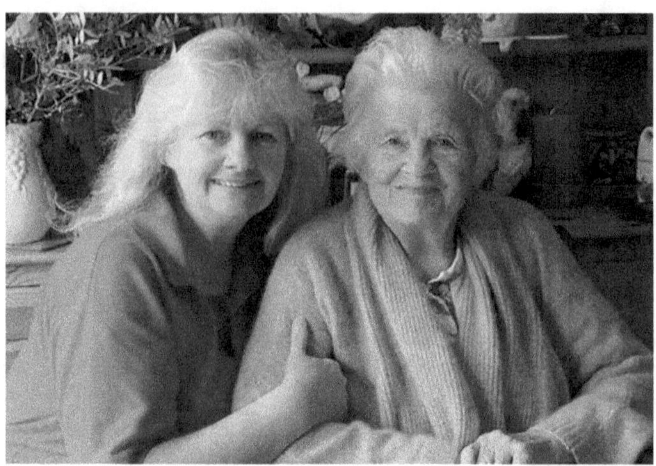

The role of the pre-existing relationship

In IDEAL, we felt it was important to consider the role of this pre-existing relationship because it can often influence how the relationship develops and changes due to dementia as people respond to the diagnosis and changes within their roles. Often within a relationship, people can have differing perspectives. These differing views may have implications later on as the dyad copes with the diagnosis. In IDEAL, for instance, we explored the perspectives of the carer and person with dementia on the well-being of the person with dementia. We found that the carer tended to describe the person's well-being less positively than the person's own rating (Wu et al., 2020). These differences in opinion could have implications for other areas of the dyad's lives. Later in the chapter, we will look at how the individual perspectives of the carer and person with dementia might influence one another's well-being.

Dementia will create some challenges even for those in a very supportive relationship. People who have been in very close relationships may find it difficult to adjust to the changes within the relationship. As will be discussed later in the chapter, a decline in quality of the relationship is not always inevitable; it is possible to still maintain a good relationship. As we discussed in Chapter 4, the relationship can be a huge source of comfort and many carers identify great strength from the relationship within their caring role (Quinn et al., 2024).

It is often assumed that caring takes place within the context of a 'good' relationship. Yet carers take on the caring role for a multitude of reasons, particularly if we think about the different types of carers. Often the caring role is perceived as a natural continuation of the relationship. In IDEAL, spouses often mentioned marital duties or vows of 'in sickness and health' (Quinn et al., 2024).

Children can see helping a parent as a form of positive 'payback' or reciprocity for previous support given (Quinn et al., 2009). However, there can be societal or cultural obligations, which means that people feel that they have little choice but to take on the caring role and may end up feeling trapped (Quinn et al., 2015). Females are more likely to be carers and changes in roles can be experienced differently by males and females. For instance, men are more likely to get help with caring (Erol et al., 2016). There may also be other practicalities that can lead to some taking on the caring role, such as a lack of financial resources to pay for formal care services. The person with dementia may have expressed their own views, preferring to be supported by family rather than formal care services (Quinn et al., 2015). Therefore, there can be quite complex reasons why a particular caring relationship is as it is.

With those possible reasons why someone might take on the caring role in mind, it is important to recognise that caring can take place within a previously 'bad' relationship; as identified by Jane, a member of the ALWAYs group: '*We should always think about relationships that weren't working before dementia, and the impact that dementia has on these relationships*'.

Not everyone will have a good relationship with their spouse/partner or parent. However, those involved in these situations may feel that they have no choice but to provide care or to draw on these individuals to help support them. For example, some people who are in a bad marriage may feel it is now impossible to divorce the other person because they have been diagnosed with dementia. For some people, these pre-existing issues will not disappear just because of the dementia and may in fact be amplified. This can lead to potential risks of abuse and safeguarding issues.

Throughout this section, the focus has been on longstanding relationships, yet a caring situation might occur in a relatively new relationship, for example in the context of a second marriage later in life. These individuals will not be able to draw on the longstanding relationship and may in fact have very different expectations from the relationship.

The impact of dementia on the relationship

Receiving a diagnosis of dementia will have an impact on a relationship; Allison, a member of the ALWAYs group, commented: '*We arrived at the diagnosis appointment as husband and wife and left as carer and person with dementia*'. This shows how dementia can alter a relationship, as one person gradually adopts the role of the carer who increasingly has to provide care for the other person, who becomes the 'care-recipient'. This means that each individual's roles and responsibilities and the overall balance of the relationship will change (Quinn et al., 2009). Consequently, the relationship may change in unpredictable ways. How each person adapts to and manages these changes will have an influence on the resulting impact on their relationship. Some dyads will cope with these changes better than others.

One of the main changes within the relationship will be in roles and responsibilities. A person with dementia we spoke to in IDEAL described some of the difficulties: '*Well I think we used to go out separately but not, not now, you know, definitely not now … I couldn't go shopping anymore. I'm terrified going out without her [the carer]*'.

Carers may feel they ought to take over tasks from the person with dementia. Some might find this challenging as they are getting involved in aspects of the person's life that are new to them. For instance, a child may know nothing about their parent's finances. It can be difficult to know how best to deal with this type of situation. The carer may feel the need to protect the person with dementia but being over-protective risks disempowering the person, who may feel they can still do things quite ably (Quinn et al., 2013). If this results in tension, the carer may feel the person does not value their help. Therefore, there needs to be a careful balance, as providing too much or too little assistance can lead to a decline in ability. Too much support can lead to the person allowing others to do things for them and losing the ability to do things for themselves. Too little support can lead to frustration, causing the person to stop trying to do things. The Living with Dementia Toolkit, introduced in Chapter 3, has a section on 'maintaining relationships' which tackles how to deal with some of these issues (IDEAL Programme, 2021).

Another aspect of the relationship that can be affected is the emotional and companionship side of the relationship. When someone develops dementia there may be changes in how they feel and behave. Carers can find this difficult to deal with, particularly if they have known the person for a long time. A child may no longer feel that they can access the same level of support from a parent with dementia. Carers may find themselves responding differently as they become more stressed. A core aspect of all relationships is communication. The person with dementia may find it more difficult to take part in conversations and may repeat what they are saying. A person with dementia we spoke to in IDEAL identified how this could be challenging for his wife: '*She's my lifeline really. I mean I feel for her at times … must be frustrating at times for a person that's close … in the vicinity all the time and if you said something and my memory has gone, it just must be frustrating as well for her at times*'. If the carer feels the person with dementia is struggling to speak, they may take over the conversation and speak on their behalf. This may affect the confidence of the person with dementia, changing the power balance in the relationship.

Relationships evolve and change

In the previous section, we considered the impact of a dementia diagnosis on the relationship. Relationships can change over time and some carers have identified a decline in the quality of their relationship over time (Quinn et al., 2012). In IDEAL, we found that the carer and the person with dementia may have very different views about the quality of the relationship, with the carer feeling much less positive about it (Rippon et al., 2020).

Relationships do evolve. ALWAYs group members recognised how their relationships had changed since the diagnosis. They commented that the roles of 'carer' and 'care-recipient' were not inevitable, and changes could be made to allow people to continue in pre-existing roles. Jane, a member of the ALWAYs group, shown in the photograph below doing a memory walk with her mother on a rainy day, felt it was important that any changes were recognised and discussed: *'My mum would remind me by saying "I'm the mum" when I took over. I cared for her and equally she cared for me. People with dementia pick up on emotions, and when I was sad, she could care for me. It was a partnership'*.

Some carers in IDEAL spoke about how, through providing care, they had noticed some improvements in their relationship with the person with dementia. This could be because they were spending more time together and had grown closer. Child carers talked about getting to know their parent better through providing care (Quinn et al., 2024).

Jane and her mother Ella on a fundraising memory walk.

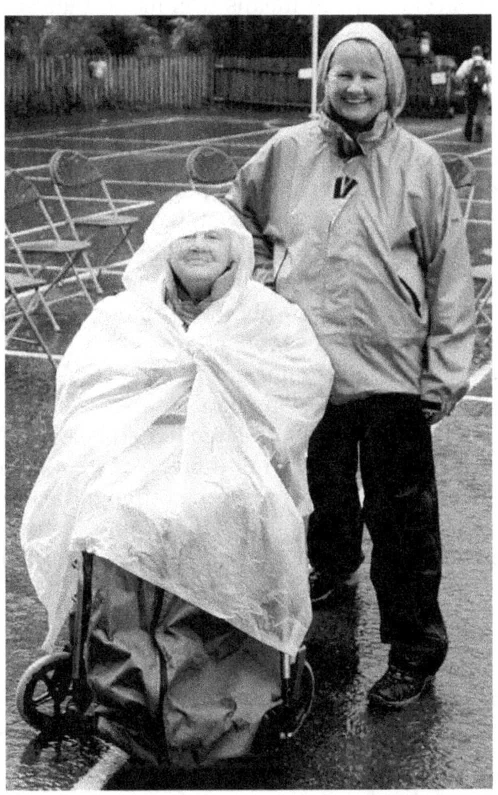

How the relationship between the carer and person with dementia can influence well-being

So far in this chapter, we have been considering the potential changes that can take place within a relationship. Why are these changes important? In IDEAL, we explored whether the quality of the relationship influenced the well-being of the person with dementia and carer. We also explored how each person might influence the other's well-being; as Keith, a member of the ALWAYs group, described: *'The person with dementia and carer are two sides of the same coin. My wife's good days are mine and vice versa'*.

Having a good relationship with the carer is important for the quality of life of people with dementia (Martyr et al., 2018). For carers, having a better pre-caring and current relationship with the person with dementia is linked to lower feelings of role captivity (feeling trapped in the caring role) and care-related stress (Quinn et al., 2012). In the IDEAL model of living well for carers, discussed in Chapter 4, we found that the quality of the carer's relationship with the person with dementia had a minor influence on whether carers were living well (Clare et al., 2022). For carers who initially had a poorer relationship with the person with dementia, well-being was more likely to decline over time.

The nature of this relationship means it is likely that each member of the dyad will have an influence on the other's well-being. In IDEAL, we found that feelings of depression in people with dementia or carers negatively influenced living well for both the person experiencing them and the other member of the dyad (Wu et al., 2021). If the carer felt depressed, this led to poorer well-being for the person with dementia and vice versa. In IDEAL, we also explored how the quality of the relationship influenced people's well-being. For both members of the dyad, the quality of the relationship influenced their own well-being. However, the carer's views on the quality of the relationship did not influence the well-being of the person with dementia and vice versa (Rippon et al., 2020). This could be because the carer and person with dementia are not completely aware of the other's views on the relationship.

In IDEAL, we also explored the influence of carers' experiences of caring on the well-being of people with dementia. Poorer well-being in people with dementia was associated with the carer feeling stressed and unsupported by other people and thinking they were not doing a very good job in their caring role. This suggests that how the carer is experiencing the caring role can have an impact on the person with dementia. What we have found in IDEAL highlights how the well-being of one member of the dyad can influence the other. This demonstrates the need to support both members of the dyad.

Transitions in the relationship

We have so far considered the types of changes that might occur within a relationship after a diagnosis of dementia. Yet there are likely to be more major changes, or transitions, in this relationship, particularly when someone's living situation changes or when dementia becomes more advanced. A person with dementia may find their situation changes if the carer is no longer able to continue in the role, for example if the carer becomes unwell. Similarly, a carer may find that the needs of the person with dementia have increased so much that they are no longer able to cope. This can lead to them seeking assistance from formal care services or deciding the person needs to move into a care home. These types of transitions can bring changes in the relationship because of the other people now involved in the care of the person with dementia.

One transitional event is that as the person's dementia progresses, they will find it harder to do things for themselves. In time, they may have difficulties recognising the carer, which can be a distressing experience. They may find it harder to speak. Yet in IDEAL, we found that there are ways of supporting communication for people with advanced dementia (Collins et al., 2022), including using photographs or objects that are meaningful to the person to encourage responses and conversation. There are also other ways of communicating that do not rely on speech, such as eye contact or a smile. Family members have described how these cues indicate that the person still recognises them (Quinn et al., 2014).

The greatest transition that can occur is the person with dementia entering into full-time care. There are many reasons that might trigger this transition. For carers it may be due to factors such as a decline in the person's abilities, their own physical health, or the person no longer recognising them (Quinn et al., 2015). This creates many changes. If the two members of the dyad had been living together, then it can be a major event to live separately. They may find that they are not as able to spend as much time together. The carer will need to adjust to being less involved in supporting the person with dementia. There will be others involved in caring who the carer will now need to engage with. Despite this, some carers will feel that they are still the person's carer and have a caring role in that person's life. Although these changes may be difficult to adjust to, there is the potential for some positive benefits. For example, it may mean that the dyad has more quality time together as the carer is less stressed because they are no longer providing a high level of hands-on care. Even if the person is in a residential home, aspects of the relationship such as affection or companionship can still be maintained. The following quote is from a gentleman I met whose wife had advanced dementia and now lived in a care home, where they would often be sitting in chairs next to each other: *'She'll lean, reach out and catches hold of my hand and hangs on. At times she lifts it up and kisses the back of my hand ... you still think well there is a connection somewhere along the line don't you?'* (Quinn et al., 2014: 263).

So what does this tell us about reconsidering living with dementia?

This chapter has focused on the relationship between the person with dementia and carer. Often these individuals get treated as separate entities, but this approach fails to take into account the impact of the relationship on patterns of interacting with one another and on individual perspectives. In IDEAL, we have shown how we need to rethink our view of this relationship. The quality of this relationship can have an impact on the well-being of the person with dementia and the carer. Over time a poor relationship can be linked to a decline in carers' well-being. We have also shown how the well-being of the carer can influence the person with dementia and vice versa. Rather than viewing the person with dementia and carer as separate entities, we need to ensure that they are supported together as a dyad.

People with dementia and carers should not be expected to manage relationship changes alone. Often the formal support provided after the diagnosis of dementia focuses on adjusting to the diagnosis, rather than on how people will adjust to any changes to their relationship. It can be difficult to change long-standing patterns of behaviour and communication, but with support beneficial changes can be made. Dyads need support to adjust to changes in the balance of roles within their relationship so that carers are not too over-protective and people with dementia do not feel disempowered. It can be tough to get that balance right and this is why people need help. Ultimately, receiving continued support to adjust to relationship changes can have long-lasting benefits for the person with dementia and their carer.

> **Reflections from the ALWAYs group**
>
> We recognised the impact of the dementia diagnosis on a relationship and how people's roles within that relationship may start to become defined by their role within a caring partnership rather than within the original relationship. We appreciated that there would be some relationships that 'weren't working' before the dementia and that this may present some challenges. We understood that transitional events, such as the person entering residential care, can lead to changes in the relationship. These transitions can lead to some positives for the relationship, such as enabling individuals to have more quality time together.
>
> We think specialist support to help with relationships should be provided. Support services should recognise dyads, rather than supporting the person with dementia and carer as separate entities. They should be cared for as part of the dyad, so the relationship itself almost becomes a third element of the partnership.

> **Key points**
>
> **Key points for people with dementia and carers**
>
> - It is important to take care of yourself; how you are feeling will influence how the other person is feeling.

- It is important to talk about changes in relationship roles; do not just let the changes happen.
- Work together to preserve the companionship aspect of your relationship.

Key points for health and social care practitioners

- Recognise that when people with dementia and carers come as dyads, you need to work with them together.
- The well-being of the person with dementia may be influencing the well-being of the carer and vice versa.
- Offer people with dementia and carers support to help them navigate any changes within their relationship.

Key points for policy-makers

- The relationship between the person with dementia and carer is at the core of the caring relationship.
- Health and social care policies should ensure that the relationship is supported.

⚑ Manifesto statement

Relationships matter: we want to be supported to maintain our relationships.

References

Clare, L., Gamble, L.D., Martyr, A., et al. (2022) 'Living well' trajectories among family caregivers of people with mild-to-moderate dementia in the IDEAL cohort, *Journals of Gerontology B: Psychological Sciences and Social Sciences*, 77(10): 1852–63.

Collins, R., Hunt, A., Quinn, C., et al. (2022) Methods and approaches for enhancing communication with people with moderate-to-severe dementia that can facilitate their inclusion in research and service evaluation: findings from the IDEAL programme, *Dementia*, 21(4): 1135–53.

Erol, R., Brooker, D. and Peel, E. (2016) The impact of dementia on women internationally: an integrative review, *Health Care for Women International*, 37(12): 1320–41.

IDEAL Programme (2021) *Setting yourself goals*, Living with Dementia Toolkit. Available at: https://livingwithdementiatoolkit.org.uk/stay-positive/maintaining-relationships/ (accessed 3 September 2024).

Martyr, A., Nelis, S.M., Quinn, C., et al. (2018) Living well with dementia: a systematic review and correlational meta-analysis of factors associated with quality of life, well-being and life satisfaction in people with dementia, *Psychological Medicine*, 48(13): 2130–39.

Quinn, C., Clare, L. and Woods, R.T. (2009) The impact of motivations and meanings on the wellbeing of caregivers of people with dementia: a systematic review, *International Psychogeriatrics*, 22(1): 43–55.

Quinn, C., Clare, L., McGuinness, T., et al. (2012) The impact of relationships, motivations, and meanings on dementia caregiving outcomes, *International Psychogeriatrics*, 24(11): 1816–26.

Quinn, C., Clare, L., McGuinness, T., et al. (2013) Negotiating the balance: the triadic relationship between spousal caregivers, people with dementia and Admiral Nurses, *Dementia* 12(5): 588–605.

Quinn, C., Clare, L., Jelley, H., et al. (2014) 'It's in the eyes': how family members and care staff understand awareness in people with severe dementia, *Aging and Mental Health*, 18(2): 260–68.

Quinn, C., Clare, L. and Woods, R.T. (2015) Balancing needs: the role of motivations, meanings and relationship dynamics in the experience of informal caregivers of people with dementia, *Dementia*, 14(2): 220–37.

Quinn, C., Toms, G., Rippon, I., et al. (2024) Positive experiences in dementia care-giving: findings from the IDEAL programme, *Ageing and Society*, 44(5): 1010–30.

Rippon, I., Quinn, C., Martyr, A., et al. (2020) The impact of relationship quality on life satisfaction and well-being in dementia caregiving dyads: findings from the IDEAL study, *Aging and Mental Health*, 24(9): 1411–20.

Wu, Y.-T., Nelis, S.M., Quinn, C., et al. (2020) Factors associated with self- and informant ratings of quality of life, well-being and life satisfaction in people with mild-to-moderate dementia: results from the Improving the experience of Dementia and Enhancing Active Life programme, *Age and Ageing*, 49(3): 446–52.

Wu, Y.-T., Clare, L. and Matthews, F.E. (2021) Relationship between depressive symptoms and capability to live well in people with dementia and their carers: results from the Improving the experience of Dementia and Enhancing Active Life (IDEAL) programme, *Aging and Mental Health*, 25(1): 38–45.

Dementia in daily life: everyday activities

Anthony Martyr, Catherine Charlwood and Linda Clare

> *Most of the things I do aren't affected by words, playing games, bowls and badminton and painting. But as soon as you meet people that's when you realize that there's anything wrong, you try to tell them about what you've been doing, well you start hitting gaps.*
>
> (A person with dementia participating in IDEAL)

In this chapter we will:

- consider the importance of being able to engage in everyday activities
- explore the potential for greater inclusion through improving public awareness and inclusive design of physical spaces and technology
- demonstrate how simple, practical strategies and assistive technology can help to compensate for difficulties and maintain involvement in activities
- show how rehabilitation practitioners and services can offer personalised support that enables people to be as independent as possible

What we do is central to who we are

Each day we all do many different things, often without even thinking about them. We get up, prepare and eat breakfast, wash and dress – all before we start whatever we have planned for that day. As we get ready, we make hundreds of small decisions, often without realising just how many choices we are making. What would it feel like if all these choices became much more difficult? What difference would it make to your life? This is a challenge that people with dementia face daily.

We tend to think about dementia mainly in terms of changes in mental abilities, but this is not the whole story. Mental skills such as memory, language, visual perception, and problem-solving underpin everything we do. Changes in mental abilities start gradually long before a diagnosis is made and increase as dementia progresses, and as they change, so does our ability to engage in and manage all the activities that make up our waking lives (Martyr et al., 2024). This is a part of living with mild-to-moderate dementia that generally receives less attention from services, even though for people with dementia themselves these changes have a profound effect.

What we do and how we spend our time is central to our sense of who we are. How we manage the many things that we need to do to look after ourselves and be involved as a member of society gives us our independence. At a basic level we wash, eat, and dress each day, but many of the things we do are more complex and rely on a wider range of abilities, such as shopping, driving, or using a mobile phone. To participate in social activities or other pastimes, we may need to draw on various abilities – reading information about the event, using the telephone or email to arrange to meet a friend, planning the journey, making our way there, and problem-solving around any disruption to the journey – before we even begin to take part in the activity itself.

What we do and how we spend our time is also centrally important for quality of life. Our systematic review showed that people with dementia who were better able to manage everyday activities rated their quality of life more positively (Martyr et al., 2018). IDEAL participants told us the same thing; being able to do everyday tasks was linked with better quality of life (Martyr et al., 2019). People feel more positive and confident if they can do the things they want and need to do and maintain a sense of independence (Kim and Shin, 2023). As we saw in Chapter 3, continuing to engage in daily activities and maintaining as much independence as possible are key priorities for people with dementia (Quinn et al., 2022b).

The impact of changes in what people can do

Changes and losses in what they can do may be distressing for people with dementia. As Keith from the ALWAYs group told us, *'There's a sadness about things you used to do – it's very hard to walk away, to have a Plan B removed'*. Another person with dementia, discussing daily routine during an IDEAL interview, said: *'I can't always do things, and that makes me so angry with me'*. Changes in abilities can lead to loss of confidence and motivation, so that people stop doing the things they used to enjoy. It can mean that people become isolated because they stop going out or meeting other people, probably leading to more rapid changes.

These changes also affect carers who provide support. It can be upsetting for them to see the person being less active, and they may be troubled if the person expresses frustration or anger. Allison from the ALWAYs group, sharing experiences for the Living with Dementia Toolkit, commented that when she gets frustrated about not being able to find the word she wants to say, '*Quite often, family will say "Are you really cross?" and you're not really cross. It's just this damn thing [dementia], really*' (IDEAL Programme, 2023a). Of course, it can be frustrating for family members, too, if the person with dementia forgets something important or takes longer to get things done, especially if they are dealing with their own stresses. This can sometimes show up as grief. As Jane from the ALWAYs group told us: '*When your loved one can't do something they've always been able to do, you feel that loss of something important*'. Family members often prioritise avoiding risk when it comes to engaging in activities outside the home. They may worry about potential accidents or incidents that could occur in unfamiliar environments. This can make it difficult to appreciate both the things the person can still do and the importance of having opportunities to enjoy activities outside the home.

There are various reasons why people with dementia and their carers may have different ideas about what the person with dementia is able to do. In IDEAL, we asked people with dementia a series of questions about their current ability to do everyday tasks like managing money, going shopping alone and making telephone calls (Martyr et al., 2019). Carers, where available, answered the same questions about how they saw the person's ability. People with dementia and carers agreed about what kinds of tasks are generally easier, such as making hot drinks, or harder, such as managing finances (Martyr et al., 2014). However, people with dementia saw themselves as better able to do these kinds of tasks than carers did (Martyr et al., 2022). We might assume that the carers know best, but in fact when we watch people with dementia doing these tasks, we find that what they are able to do corresponds better with their own estimates of their ability than with the carers' estimates (Martyr and Clare, 2018). If family members underestimate what the person can do, they may be more inclined to take over doing things that the person finds difficult. They may believe they are being helpful, or perhaps it is just easier or quicker, and less stressful, to do the task themselves than to involve the person with dementia. Taking over might sometimes be necessary, but in general it is counterproductive as the person is likely to lose abilities more rapidly. To maintain abilities, we may need to think about doing things in different ways or with more support, but it is important for people with dementia to keep doing as much as possible.

Discussions about dementia often centre on what people cannot do or have difficulty doing, assuming that nothing can be done about changes in ability to manage everyday activities. The discussion should focus instead on strengths and retained abilities and how these can be supported. While people may need help and support to overcome difficulties, this can often be built around what someone can still do. We made a video for the Living with Dementia Toolkit which gives some examples of this (IDEAL Programme, 2021b). For instance, instead of doing someone's shopping for them, could you accompany them and offer support if needed, perhaps by reminding them to check the shopping list? Rather than making a telephone call on someone's behalf, could you dial the number, but then pass the phone over to them? This shift in mindset is fundamental in promoting a personalised approach that enables people with dementia to live as independently as possible for as long as possible. It also encourages a more positive and empowering perspective for everyone involved and produces opportunities for maintaining a sense of purpose and fulfilment in the daily lives of people with dementia (Kitwood, 1997).

It is certainly true that dementia symptoms such as forgetfulness make it harder to do things, but this is only one part of the story. There are other reasons why engaging in activities might be difficult for people with dementia. Some of these are connected to how people with dementia and those supporting them react. We mentioned loss of confidence and motivation earlier, and difficulty with activities can make people feel anxious or depressed. These reactions, while completely understandable, tend to make things harder, so helping to navigate them could reduce that element of extra challenge. We look at this in more detail in Chapter 9. Other reasons are nothing to do with the person or carer but have more to do with the world around us; we look at this in more detail in Chapter 5. Unhelpful social interactions can be hurtful and can result in withdrawing from social contact to avoid feelings of shame or embarrassment. One person with dementia talked about how people they regarded as friends started to distance themselves once they were diagnosed with dementia. As well as being hurtful, it limited their opportunities to get involved in things and left them feeling isolated. People we know or encounter in public places may not understand dementia and may be impatient or critical. More generally, though, the world we live in is complex and typically not designed for people experiencing any kind of difficulty. As a society, we now expect that buildings have ramps and lifts so that people who cannot use stairs can still get inside. We have not yet taken on board the idea of designing or adapting environments and services to include people with 'hidden' difficulties.

Identifying and addressing barriers

Thinking about dementia in this way opens up a new perspective. Rather than focusing on disease, impairment, and cure, we find ourselves in the realm of disability. This approach is more optimistic, enabling us to identify and change barriers that exclude people with dementia and suggest practical steps that can make a difference. Considering dementia as a disease helps us understand the brain changes involved in each type of dementia and find ways of tackling these, but thinking this way can sometimes fall short in terms of addressing the needs of people living with the condition here and now. Broadening our viewpoint and thinking about the ways in which relationships and environments shape the experience of living with dementia reminds us that these aspects can be either enabling or disabling.

The ability to engage in activities and participate in society is influenced not just by biological features but also by the person's physical, psychological, and individual characteristics, and by the social and environmental context. This is expressed in the biopsychosocial model of human functioning (World Health Organization, 2001). Influential thinkers about quality of life for people with dementia have similarly emphasised the importance of social context (Kitwood, 1997) and the intersection between environmental quality, psychological well-being, and 'behavioural competence', or the ability to engage in activities (Lawton, 1994). Drawing on this way of thinking encourages us to reconsider possibilities for enabling people with dementia from two perspectives: contextual and personal (Clare, 2017). The contextual dimension focuses on environments and relationships. We have looked in detail at social connections in Chapter 5 and close relationships in Chapter 6, so here we will think about the environments in which people with dementia live.

Making the environments we live in more inclusive

Acknowledging the challenges that environments can pose, the move to create dementia-friendly communities promotes inclusivity and understanding of the condition. This helps reduce stigma by raising awareness among community members and organisations, and providing education on how to address the needs of people with dementia (Quinn et al., 2022a). Adapting public spaces to be more accessible can greatly enhance the ability of people with dementia to participate in community activities (Quinn et al., 2022a). When we spoke to people with dementia and carers in North Wales as part of our opera project, many people cited nature and the outdoors as good features of their local communities (IDEAL Programme, 2023b). They mentioned tarmacked paths, flat surfaces, and the availability of accessible toilets as things they needed: they focused on the ways in which the outdoors could be made accessible for them. One effective way to create a more dementia-friendly town centre is to have effective signage. Clear, simple, and visually distinct signs can greatly help people with dementia to find their way around (Van Schaik et al., 2008). Pedestrianised areas that channel people away from busy roads, and enclosed shopping centres offering protection from extremes of weather, are also helpful (Blackman et al., 2007), especially if they include accessible toilets. Making environments more inclusive for people with dementia is discussed in more detail in Chapter 5

While most people know that dementia can cause memory problems, fewer are aware of the many other ways in which changes in the brain can affect people's ability to engage in activities. For example, people with dementia can experience sensory changes that affect how they perceive the world around them. This makes navigating certain environments tricky. When we discussed this with the ALWAYs group, they talked about the way in which dementia affects visual perception:

ALLISON: *I can be uncertain about surfaces – I'm not sure where they are. I tap my foot even if I know logically it's there. The way a floor is laid out can make me think it's at a strange angle. 'Is that flat?' I ask my husband.*

JANE: *For my mum, the carpet could change colour, so darker carpets or patterns could be challenging. A small change to something visually could have a big impact – a haircut could mean she didn't recognise someone. Glass balustrades were a nightmare – my mum didn't see them.*

ALLISON: *Glass is the worst!*

Understanding these kinds of challenges and making architects and designers aware of them creates opportunities for adapting plans and designs to be more inclusive. If managers of hotels and other public venues know about the disabling effects of darker or patterned flooring, this might encourage them to choose something more neutral instead. Adaptations of this kind can help to combat the risk of people with dementia experiencing a prematurely 'shrinking world' (Duggan et al., 2008).

Similarly, people with dementia can find it harder to process information and solve problems quickly. Many of the interactions we have when out and about are not with other people at all but with computer-driven machines of one kind or another. Purchasing a ticket to use public transport often means interacting with a ticket machine that provides little guidance about how to operate it, requires quick choices, and is unforgiving if the wrong button is pressed. This can be frustrating or off-putting for anyone but could deter people with dementia from travelling altogether. More user-friendly alternatives that offer the chance to talk to and get help from a real person are still needed. Many of us now use automated teller machines (ATMs) – commonly referred to as cashpoints – to obtain cash and deposit funds. One of the banners in 'The Unfurlings' project that we introduced in Chapter 3 focused on the difficulties people with dementia experience in using these. The Face it Together peer support group created a banner showing on one side the ways in which people with dementia struggle with ATMs, and on the other the rewards of managing this successfully, such as being able to visit outdoor places. This highlights the benefits of enabling people with dementia to manage these kinds of activities: being able to use a ticket machine could improve self-confidence and mood, and the subsequent activity might take place with other people, reinforcing social connections and allowing the person with dementia to enjoy time outdoors. The Face it Together group wanted to encourage the companies concerned with ATMs to talk to people living with dementia and find out about the problems they experience, and then use this information to improve their systems and products (Beesley et al., 2020). This is why the banner shows the mantra 'Involve, Inform, Improve' (see Figure 7.1).

Figure 7.1: Face it Together Bradford banner 'Involve, Inform, Improve'.

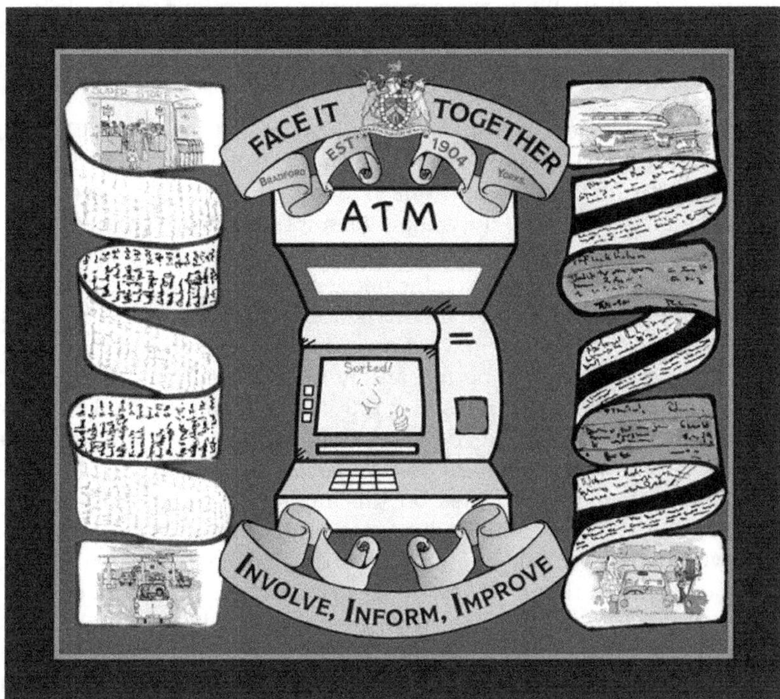

Strategies for managing daily challenges

At the personal level, people with dementia and their families often find ways to manage everyday challenges. They focus on the person's strengths and abilities. Sometimes it is possible to simplify activities or break down more complex tasks into a series of smaller steps that are more manageable and reduce demands on memory or planning ability. Practical changes could include labelling drawers and cupboards to indicate what is inside them or creating a set of simple instructions for operating a kitchen appliance. Small changes like this may seem trivial but make it possible to continue doing tasks rather than having to depend on someone else. These can make a big difference to a person's sense of worth and well-being. Using a whiteboard or diary to list activities for the day and crossing these off as they happen can help with keeping track of the daily schedule. Sometimes activities must be done in a different way. For example, if reading becomes difficult, listening to an audio book might be a workable alternative.

These kinds of adaptations often involve the use of assistive technology. This term covers any devices that help people deal with everyday activities, from low-tech aids like walking sticks to high-tech ones like smart phones. Most people with dementia who took part in IDEAL used at least one form of assistive technology or adaptation to assist them in their daily activities (Henderson et al., 2019). While some more high-tech options can be difficult for people with dementia to use, there are often simplified versions available, like featurephones or video-call systems that help people stay in touch with family and friends.

Sometimes it can be difficult to know how to get started with thinking about adaptations and ways of compensating for challenges. It can also be difficult to make further adaptations if dementia symptoms worsen. Episodes of ill-health, especially if a stay in hospital is involved, can affect what people are able to do and require new strategies to support recovery. In these situations, professional help may be needed. This is called reablement or rehabilitation. Practitioners take a holistic look at the person's strengths and difficulties and overall situation, find out what the person wants or needs to achieve, improve, or manage better, and help to identify and implement the strategies that can make this possible (Rahja and Thuesen, 2023). The World Health Organization (WHO) has developed a package of rehabilitation interventions for people with dementia (see WHO, 2023). Cognitive rehabilitation for people with dementia focuses on the impact of changes in mental (or 'cognitive') abilities on activity and participation. Practitioners work collaboratively with people with dementia to identify clear, realistic goals and build strategies to achieve them. These goals are personal and reflect that person's preferences and needs. The strategies are equally personal. The same activity might be difficult for different reasons depending on the person. If the goal is to bake a cake, one person might be too anxious to get started, another might have trouble assembling ingredients, another might have trouble concentrating and following the recipe, and another might forget to remove the cake from the oven and burn it. By understanding the specific challenges, the practitioner can identify the strategies most likely to help. These strategies could involve compensating for difficulties, adapting the person's environment, introducing assistive technologies, or using enhanced learning methods such as expanding rehearsal and mnemonics to enable people to learn or re-learn information.

Evidence shows that by using this approach we can enable people to reach their goals and improve how they manage the chosen activities (Kudlicka et al., 2023). This may enable people to continue living in their own homes for longer (Amieva et al., 2016). Carol, living with dementia, describes how she found cognitive rehabilitation helpful:

> *I started the course three months after my diagnosis. The first thing we have done was come up with some of the problems I was struggling with on a daily basis and from there we whittled it down to the two major things I was struggling with ... As well as benefiting from the specific strategies I developed as part of the therapy, I also developed a set of tools and techniques that I can now apply to pretty much any problem I come across. GREAT Cognitive Rehabilitation has helped (and is still helping me, 2 years on!) to find ways to tackle the problems that arise with everyday tasks.*

For people who want to try this approach the My Life, My Goals self-help resource offers a step-by-step approach to identifying and reaching goals using the principles of cognitive rehabilitation (IDEAL Programme, 2021a) (see Figure 7.2). For practitioners, there is an e-learning course available to help develop the skills to support people through the cognitive rehabilitation approach; practitioners working in the UK National Health Service can access it on the NHS Learning Hub (https://learninghub.nhs.uk/), and those outside the UK can find it on the GREAT cognitive rehabilitation website (https://sites.google.com/exeter.ac.uk/great-cr/home).

Figure 7.2: The My Life, My Goals self-management resource.

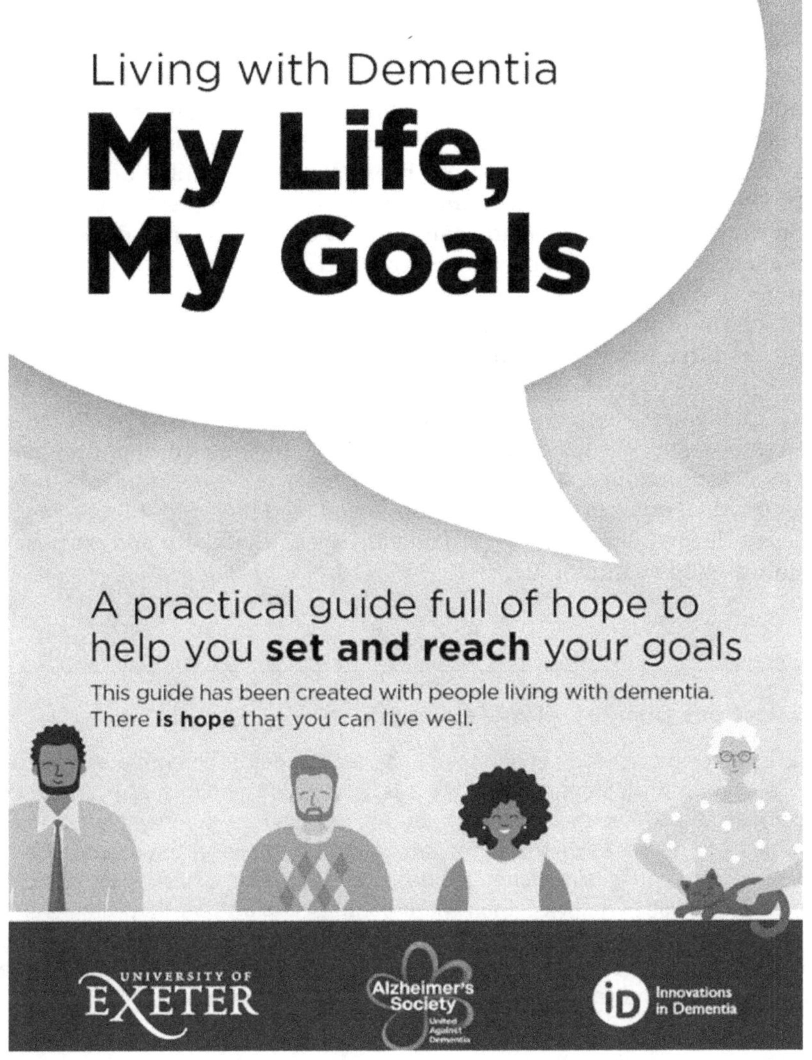

So what does this tell us about reconsidering living with dementia?

What we do is important. When thinking about living with dementia, we need to place more emphasis on what people do and the activities they engage in. This is a crucial aspect of people's lives and one that is closely linked to experiencing a good quality of life. There are three main aspects that we need to reconsider.

Rather than thinking about impairments, we need to think about strengths and abilities. We need to focus on what people can do rather than what they cannot do. We need to find ways of enabling them to make full use of the abilities they have, even if this takes longer or is less convenient. We need to challenge assumptions about what people might be able to do and be creative in thinking about opportunities to try new activities and things that might bring pleasure and a sense of purpose.

Rather than allowing people to be excluded, we need to understand the ways in which environments can be disabling and what can be done to change this and create a more enabling context. From provision of facilities in outdoor environments to design of furnishings and new technologies, considering the way in which the decisions made can serve to enable and include people with dementia will produce environments and surroundings that work better for everyone.

We need a change of mindset about how we support people with dementia. We need to encourage people to adapt to the impact of changes in mental abilities on what they do and get involved in, and find helpful strategies to get around challenges, so they can stay involved and maintain as much independence as possible. We need to enable and encourage services and individual practitioners to adopt a personalised approach that supports people to reach their individual goals and stay active, involved, and included. Embracing such an approach can help people with dementia live with dignity and purpose and maintain a good quality of life.

Reflections from the ALWAYs group

The chapter provides practical solutions to everyday problems encountered while living with dementia. We think it is worth highlighting that even basic, everyday tasks, such as making a cup of tea, can be surprisingly complex and lead to distress when they go wrong. These tasks, often repeated and familiar, can cause significant upset and feelings of being useless when difficulties arise – more so than more complex tasks – as they emphasise feelings of inadequacy in people who have performed these tasks their entire lives. The chapter offers valuable and accessible information for both people with dementia and carers to help manage these challenges.

Key points

Key points for people with dementia and carers

- Focus on your strengths and abilities rather than on what you cannot do.
- Think about how to adapt your surroundings and activities to make things more manageable.
- Establish consistent routines and use visual reminders such as labels to help remember what needs to be done.

Key points for health and social care practitioners

- Support people with dementia in ways that are personalised and tailored to individual abilities and preferences.
- Learn how to help people with dementia and their families develop strategies for managing everyday activities.
- Campaign to make indoor and outdoor public places accessible and dementia-friendly.

Key points for policy-makers

- Support initiatives that promote personalisation of care and support.
- Consider the relevance and value of reablement and rehabilitative interventions.
- Find ways to make public spaces and buildings accessible for people with 'hidden' disabilities like dementia.

 **Manifesto statement**

We want to be encouraged and enabled to do as much as we can.

References

Amieva, H., Robert, P.H., Grandoulier, A.S., et al. (2016) Group and individual cognitive therapies in Alzheimer's disease: the ETNA3 randomized trial, *International Psychogeriatrics*, 28(5): 707–17.

Beesley, I., Hall, M., Husband, T., et al. (2020) *The Unfurlings: Banners for Hope and Change*. York: Darkroom Press.

Blackman, T., Van Schaik, P. and Martyr, A. (2007) Outdoor environments for people with dementia: an exploratory study using virtual reality, *Ageing and Society*, 27(6): 811–25.

Clare, L. (2017) Rehabilitation for people living with dementia: a practical framework of positive support, *PLoS Medicine*, 14(3): e1002245. Available at: https://doi.org/10.1371/journal.pmed.1002245.

Duggan, S., Blackman, T., Martyr, A., et al. (2008) The impact of early dementia on outdoor life: a 'shrinking world'?, *Dementia*, 7(2): 191–204.

Henderson, C., Knapp, M., Nelis, S.M., et al. (2019) Use and costs of services and unpaid care for people with mild-to-moderate dementia: baseline results from the IDEAL cohort study, *Alzheimer's and Dementia: Translational Research and Clinical Interventions*, 5(1): 685–96.

IDEAL Programme (2021a) *Setting yourself goals*, Living with Dementia Toolkit. Available at: livingwithdementiatoolkit.org.uk/keep-a-sense-of-purpose/setting-yourself-goals/ (accessed 3 September 2024).

IDEAL Programme (2021b) *Why are everyday activities important?* Available at: www.youtube.com/watch?v=dRTik0MPYos (accessed 3 September 2024).

IDEAL Programme (2023a) *The ALWAYs group answers the opera cast's questions: part 2.* Available at: www.youtube.com/watch?v=ciwLfP4Ryvs (accessed 3 September 2024).

IDEAL Programme (2023b) *How can we improve the experience of living with dementia? A community workshop*, University of Exeter, Exeter.

Kim, J. and Shin, N. (2023) Development of the 'living well' concept for older people with dementia, *BMC Geriatrics*, 23(1): 611. Available at: https://doi.org/10.1186/s12877-023-04304-3.

Kitwood, T. (1997) *Dementia Reconsidered: The Person Comes First*. Buckingham: Open University Press.

Kudlicka, A., Martyr, A., Bahar-Fuchs, A., et al. (2023) Cognitive rehabilitation for people with mild to moderate dementia, *Cochrane Database of Systematic Reviews*, 6(6): CD013388. Available at: https://doi.org/10.1002/14651858.CD013388.pub2.

Lawton, M.P. (1994) Quality of life in Alzheimer disease, *Alzheimer Disease and Associated Disorders*, 8(suppl 3): 138–50.

Martyr, A. and Clare, L. (2018) Awareness of functional ability in people with early-stage dementia, *International Journal of Geriatric Psychiatry*, 33(1): 31–38.

Martyr, A., Nelis, S.M. and Clare, L. (2014) Predictors of perceived functional ability in early-stage dementia: self-ratings, informant ratings and discrepancy scores, *International Journal of Geriatric Psychiatry*, 29(8): 852–62.

Martyr, A., Nelis, S.M., Quinn, C., et al. (2018) Living well with dementia: a systematic review and correlational meta-analysis of factors associated with quality of life, well-being and life satisfaction in people with dementia, *Psychological Medicine*, 48(13): 2130–39.

Martyr, A., Nelis, S.M., Quinn, C., et al. (2019) The relationship between perceived functional difficulties and the ability to live well with mild-to-moderate dementia: findings from the IDEAL programme, *International Journal of Geriatric Psychiatry*, 34(8): 1251–61.

Martyr, A., Gamble, L.D., Nelis, S.M., et al. (2022) Predictors of awareness of functional ability in people with dementia: the contribution of personality, cognition, and neuropsychiatric symptoms. Findings from the IDEAL programme, *Dementia and Geriatric Cognitive Disorders*, 51(3): 221–32.

Martyr, A., Ravi, M., Gamble, L.D., et al. (2024) Trajectories of cognitive and perceived functional decline in people with dementia. Findings from the IDEAL programme, *Alzheimer's and Dementia*, 20(1): 410–20.

Quinn, C., Hart, N., Henderson, C., et al. (2022a) Developing supportive local communities: perspectives from people with dementia and caregivers participating in the IDEAL programme, *Journal of Aging and Social Policy*, 34(6): 839–59.

Quinn, C., Pickett, J.A., Litherland, R., et al. (2022b) Living well with dementia: what is possible and how to promote it, *International Journal of Geriatric Psychiatry*, 37(1). Available at: https://doi.org/10.1002/gps.5627.

Rahja, M. and Thuesen, J. (2023) Reablement and dementia, in T. Rostgaard, J. Parsons and H. Tuntland (eds) *Reablement in Long-Term Care for Older People*. Bristol: Bristol University Press/Policy Press.

Van Schaik, P., Martyr, A., Blackman, T., et al. (2008) Involving persons with dementia in the evaluation of outdoor environments, *Cyberpsychology and Behavior*, 11(4): 415–24.

World Health Organization (WHO) (2001) *International Classification of Functioning, Disability, and Health: ICF*. Geneva: WHO.

World Health Organization (WHO) (2023) *Package of interventions for rehabilitation. Module 3: Neurological conditions*. Geneva: WHO. Available at: https://www.who.int/publications/i/item/9789240071131.

Health matters: comfort and discomfort

Serena Sabatini and Jeanette Thom

(A person with dementia participating in IDEAL)

In this chapter we will:

- explain what IDEAL tells us about physical health and physical activity in people with dementia
- discuss the extra challenges that living with one or more additional health conditions pose for people with dementia
- think about the additional difficulties created when both the person with dementia and the person supporting them have other health conditions

What do we mean by physical health and physical activity?

To enable people with dementia to live as well as possible, it is not enough to help them manage their dementia symptoms. We need to think about the whole person. As previous chapters explain, many things contribute to living well with dementia. In this chapter, we focus on the physical side of living well: physical health and how it can be maintained or improved by staying active and doing physical activity.

In IDEAL, when we first met the participants, we asked them about their overall health and about what other health conditions they had. Other health conditions include things like diabetes, cancer, or heart disease. We asked about things that affect overall health, including diet and appetite, eyesight, hearing, sleep, falls, drinking alcohol, smoking, and physical activity. We defined physical activity not just as sport and structured exercise but as anything and everything that keeps people moving. This could be gardening, housework, going for a walk, or stretching in a seated position. You can see a summary of what people told us in Figure 8.1.

Figure 8.1: Health and physical activity among people with dementia in IDEAL.

Indicators of health	Findings among people with dementia participating in IDEAL
Subjective evaluation of one's health	15% said they had very poor or poor health 25% said they had fair health 60% said they had good, very good or excellent health
Smoking	95% were non-smokers,50% were ex-smokers
Sleep	15% reported poor sleep
Eyesight	7% reported poor eyesight
Hearing	6% reported poor hearing
Appetite	85% had normal appetite
Sense of smell	13% had experinced a change in their sense of smell in the previous year
Sense of taste	18% had experinced a change in their sense of taste in the previous year
Number of falls	46% had fallen at least once in the previous year
Alcohol intake	53% reported drinking alcohol
Medications	97% were taking at least one medication,the average was five medications
Other health conditions	70% had at least one other health condition
Physical inactivity	75% were physically inactive

A holistic picture of health

We asked the IDEAL participants to judge their health based on a simple question: 'Overall, how would you rate your health in the past four weeks?' Nearly two-thirds said their health was either good or excellent. The remainder said their health was fair or poor. When we looked at the various things that are linked to overall health, in many ways people were doing well. Almost all the participants with dementia were not smoking, although half of them had smoked in the past. Most were able to see well, either with or without glasses. Most had a good appetite. This was quite a positive picture, but it was not the whole story.

There were two aspects of poor health that affected most of the people with dementia we spoke with. First, at the beginning of the IDEAL study, three-quarters of the participants with dementia lived with at least one additional health condition (Nelis et al., 2019). In this respect, they were similar to people of the same age who do not have dementia. Some had as many as nine conditions, but the largest group, about half, had one to two other conditions. One in three had arthritis, more than one in three had high blood pressure, and more than one in ten had diabetes or chest problems. The older people were, the more likely they were to have other health conditions. Almost all were taking at least one type of medication, with some taking as many as five types. Two years later, the proportion of people with dementia with at least one additional health condition was even higher, at 88 per cent (Sabatini et al., 2024). Second, both at the beginning of the IDEAL study and two years later, about three-quarters of the participants with dementia did almost no physical activity.

In the rest of this chapter, we discuss the challenges created by living with multiple illnesses and poor mobility. We consider what we can do to address the health issues people with dementia may have and what can help people stay as active and healthy as possible.

Not just dementia: other health conditions

Having additional health conditions makes things harder for both the person with dementia and those who support them. This is particularly true when people with dementia have health conditions such as arthritis that cause pain, limit their ability to move around, and can reduce their independence. Around four in ten had pain and found their mobility was limited, and one in three said that this affected their usual activities. Sometimes these other conditions can seem more of a problem than dementia. As one IDEAL participant living with dementia said: '*Life's not that bad really, you get a bit fed up because of the arthritis I think, I've often said I think the arthritis is more of a problem than the dementia*'. As we saw in Chapter 2, when we talked to people living with undiagnosed dementia, they were more concerned about physical health problems, mobility difficulties, and sensory impairments, and found these had more of an impact on their lives than memory and other cognitive difficulties.

When people have both dementia and other health conditions, two unwanted scenarios may occur. On the one hand, doctors may pay more attention to the dementia and wrongly attribute other symptoms to that. This might mean that another illness goes undiagnosed, or that the person gets the wrong treatment. This is frustrating for the person with dementia, as they can feel they are not listened to:

> *Everything I try to talk to my doctor about they claim it's 'dementia' and sometimes I have to point out 'no, I've hurt my knee – that's nothing to do with my dementia!' Before I was diagnosed, the doctors tried to explain everything with the menopause: woman of a certain age, it must be the menopause!*
>
> (Allison, ALWAYs group member)

On the other hand, doctors may pay more attention to other health conditions than to dementia. This could be because they know more about another condition. People with dementia are typically looked after by doctors and other practitioners who are not specialists in dementia and who have received limited training about the condition (Koch et al., 2010). Sometimes this can lead to them unintentionally prescribing medications or combinations of medication that are unsuitable for someone with dementia (Delgado et al., 2020). Chris, a person living with dementia, found that his doctors tended to focus on his other health conditions. Responding to Allison's situation, he commented:

> *I'm the complete opposite. Given that dementia is the biggest [challenge], it's really hard to get the conversation going about dementia. With my diabetes, they're really good – getting blood tests, really proactive. Same with cardiovascular stuff. Then I have to remind them 'we haven't talked about my dementia yet'.*
>
> (Chris, ALWAYs group member)

Some of these issues arise because healthcare systems are generally set up to deal with single problems as they occur. This can work well in many cases, particularly for younger, fitter individuals, but it is not helpful when people have multiple health conditions, and especially chronic conditions such as dementia. Here, both good communication between all of the practitioners involved in a person's care and continuity of care, for example by seeing the same doctor or specialist at each visit, are vitally important. Despite growing awareness of the value of a proactive, rounded, and holistic approach that considers the whole person and addresses 'what matters' to the individual, and the fact that practitioners generally want to work in this way, it is difficult to achieve given demands on services and constraints on time and funding:

> *You don't get multiagency meetings for people with dementia in the way you do for children. Hospitals – General Practitioners – Memory Assessment Services: they're not talking to each other. They don't know you as a person, they get to know you as 'the pain in the leg'.*
>
> (Keith, ALWAYs group member)

When it comes to health, people with dementia want to be considered as a *'complete being'* (Chris, ALWAYs group member). The innovative approach taken by High Weald Lewes Havens Clinical Commissioning Group in Sussex, UK (Box 8.1), shows that, if the will is there, it is possible to redesign systems to make this possible.

Box 8.1: The Golden Ticket

From 2012 to 2020, High Weald Lewes Havens Clinical Commissioning Group (now NHS Sussex) planned and monitored the provision of health and social care to its local population, which includes a large proportion of people with dementia. Recognising that people with dementia were not receiving adequate care and often appeared in acute and emergency settings in an avoidable poor state of health, the CCG looked at available evidence and best practice and consulted patients, carers, and providers of statutory and voluntary services to find out how things could be improved. As a result, they designed the holistic Dementia Golden Ticket model of care to truly support people to live well with dementia. This combined, proactive model could be adopted by any practice. The 'Golden Ticket' identified people with dementia and those who support them in a non-stigmatising way and ensures their needs are prioritised. Key features were that the service, led by the primary care team with close involvement of, and communication with, specialists in secondary care, ensured that all staff in the primary care team received training about dementia, that people with dementia and carers had access to regular clinics held by a general practitioner with a special interest in dementia where additional time is allowed for appointments, and that the primary care team had strong connections with local voluntary groups, meaning that not only can people be linked in with social activities but also any health concerns could be identified and acted on quickly. In evaluation of this model, alongside positive feedback from patients and those who support them, there was a 25 per cent reduction in emergency hospital admissions and visits to accident and emergency services, a 15 per cent reduction in falls, and in several cases medication prescription was improved. The general practitioners both had better quality consultations with people and experienced fewer demands on their time overall. The evaluation of the service has informed current ways of working in Sussex.

A downward spiral

Poor health leads to many challenges in people's lives. In IDEAL, people with dementia who had more additional health conditions were more likely to have moderate or severe mobility problems, to be in pain, to find it hard to care for themselves, and to need help with daily activities such as cooking (Nelis et al., 2019). These difficulties, and often the consequent need to stop driving, made it harder to get out and about and meet family and friends, and meant that people were more likely to feel lonely and depressed, potentially creating a vicious cycle with increasingly negative effects. This probably goes a long way towards explaining why people with more health conditions rated their quality of life and well-being less positively than those with fewer health conditions (Sabatini et al., 2024). People with dementia who had poor eyesight, poor hearing, low appetite, poor sleep, or who had fallen at least once in the previous year, also rated their quality of life more negatively than others. People with poorer health generally continued to make the same low ratings over time. This highlights how important it is to address all the healthcare needs people with dementia have so they can continue doing things and live as well as possible. As we discussed in Chapter 7, rehabilitation (sometimes referred to as reablement or restorative care) is a goal-oriented, holistic healthcare approach that focuses on enabling people to function as well as possible in the ways that matter to them (Poulos et al., 2017). In relation to physical health, goals might relate to maintaining or improving mobility, preventing falls, managing pain, improving diet, or reviewing medications. Planning how to address a goal in the physical health domain could involve a team of practitioners with specialist skills, such as physiotherapists, occupational therapists, nurses, or doctors.

Psychological comfort despite physical discomfort

In the IDEAL living well map, which we discussed in Chapter 1, physical health is one of the life domains that influences emotions and how people feel about themselves, which is strongly linked in turn to whether they see themselves as living well. Being physically unwell, experiencing pain, or difficulty moving about, heightens the need for comfort (Kitwood, 1997). Comfort means closeness and warmth and promotes the kind of inner strength and resources that help with facing the challenges illnesses can bring. We need to make sure that we both address physical discomfort as far as possible and enable people with dementia to experience psychological comfort even where some physical discomfort remains.

Why is it important that carers are healthy, too?

Nearly three-quarters of the carers participating in IDEAL had at least one health condition at the start of the study, as we discussed in Chapter 4, and this proportion increased over time. More than half of the carers were physically inactive. Carers' own physical limitations and discomfort can affect their ability to provide personal care and engage in social and physical activities with the person with dementia. As a carer said, to provide support to a person with dementia, carers have '*to stay fit and well in a whole variety of ways*' (David, ALWAYs group member). As carers' own health challenges and the support needs of the person with dementia increase, carers in IDEAL told us how these situations lead to worry about the uncertainty and unpredictability of the future, the healthcare needs of the person with dementia, their ability to continue providing care, the support available from healthcare services, and whether they can afford to pay for home care (Hillman et al., 2023). Challenges related to individuals' health can contribute to decisions to move the person with dementia temporarily or permanently to residential care, again with significant financial consequences.

Poor health for people with dementia and, where available, their carers can result in cumulative challenges that may not be fully recognised by health and social care services. Figure 8.2 illustrates the way in which a combination of low physical activity, multiple health conditions, and other health issues may lead to worse health for both people with dementia and those who support them. This has practical and financial consequences for them and increases demand on overstretched health and social care services. Proactively addressing health challenges with a preventive approach and increasing physical activity levels can help to promote better health.

Figure 8.2: Addressing cumulative health challenges for people with dementia and their carers.

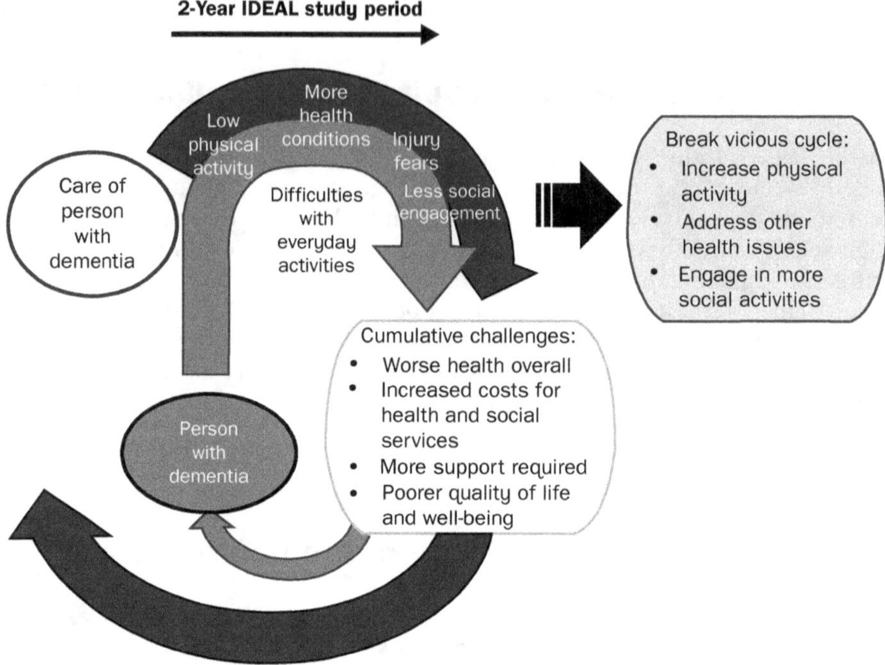

The importance of physical activity for people with dementia

Physical activity is important for everyone and we know that many people around the world, especially older people, do not undertake enough physical activity to gain the benefits it offers (Russell, 2024). Most of the people with dementia and carers taking part in IDEAL did little physical activity. This is worrying, because physical activity can help people with dementia to stay as healthy, fit, and independent as possible, and avoid falls. Physical activity also has other benefits, including improving mood, self-confidence and well-being, and providing opportunities for social contact (Nuzum et al., 2020). In IDEAL, people with dementia who were doing more physical activity had better well-being and felt more positive about their overall health than those who were physically inactive (Wu et al., 2020). One carer participating in IDEAL told us: '*I think we have coped fairly well by continuing to exercise daily*'.

Recommended activity levels are 150 minutes per week of moderate-intensity aerobic activity, such as brisk walking or swimming, or 75 minutes of vigorous-intensity activity such as jogging, ideally with exercises to increase muscle strength and balance added on two or more days a week (World Health Organization, 2020). This may seem a lot but when translated, for example, into a brisk 20-minute walk each day and a twice-weekly keep-fit class or equivalent, it sounds more manageable. Often there are local group classes for older adults run by experienced staff or online classes/recordings that can be done at home at your own pace (perhaps with a carer). The important message, though, is that adding even a small amount of exercise is beneficial, so people should not be put off if they feel these recommendations are unachievable. Almost everyone can do something to increase their activity levels and whatever they are able to do will be worthwhile.

One reason why many IDEAL participants were not physically active could be that two in five already had mobility problems that could make exercise uncomfortable or painful. Fear of falling could be another reason for avoiding physical activity. About half the IDEAL participants had fallen at least once in the previous year and many of them more than once. A carer commented from her own experience that: *'Exercise and taking to it especially after surgery is really hard because you have every reason not to do it – getting well, not wanting to injure yourself'* (Julia, ALWAYs group member). It is important that activity is tailored to a person's capabilities, and this is where professional advice and guidance from knowledgeable health and social care practitioners can be valuable. As we mentioned above, reablement programmes may help to address some of these concerns and ensure people know what they can safely do. As people's strengths and capabilities change over time, exercise choices may need to be adapted or changed. Long walks may be possible in the early stages of living with dementia, but over time the distance may need to be reduced and the pace slowed, and more support for walking introduced. If walking is not possible, seated stretching exercises or activities can be substituted.

People are more likely to be physically active when they have access to suitable opportunities and indoor and outdoor facilities and environments (Evans, 2024; Owen et al., 2024), including blue (coast, rivers, lakes) and green (parks, gardens, woodland) areas, as we described in Chapter 5. Having a dog encourages people to keep walking; IDEAL participants who cared for a pet dog walked more than those who did not (Opdebeeck et al., 2021). For many, companionship is also important, and activity groups are popular options. These include walking and activity groups (see, for example, Ramblers, n.d.; Lutheran Community Services Northwest, n.d.; Alzheimer's Western Australia, n.d.), gardening groups (see, for example, Sensory Trust, n.d.; Labirinto Cooperativa Sociale, n.d.; Fielder and Marsh, 2021), and dance classes (see, for example, Scottish Ballet, n.d.). The Living with Dementia Toolkit has a 'Stay Active' section containing a wealth of ideas about how to become active, examples of what others living with dementia have found useful, and where to find suitable exercise options (IDEAL Programme, 2021). As dementia progresses, green care farms in the Netherlands, Norway and Japan offer a more active alternative to traditional day care programmes, specialist riding centres in the United States offer opportunities to interact with and in some cases ride horses, and care home residents, who rarely get out into nature, benefit for example from group visits to woodlands (Collins et al., 2023). Community groups, voluntary sector providers, and businesses in the outdoor visitor economy who provide access to spaces and activities all have a role to play in ensuring accessible provision for people with dementia (Page et al., 2023). Increasing awareness of what appropriate services are available in local communities and online will enable more people with dementia and carers to benefit. Improving transportation to ensure that even those living in rural areas can access groups is also essential. Funding and commitment are vital to support these new and innovative initiatives.

So what does this tell us about rethinking living with dementia?

Our research made us realise that we need to rethink three issues. First, health systems need to move away from a structure where a single health condition or issue is treated at a time and towards an arrangement where all the healthcare needs of the person with dementia are treated holistically.

Second, we need to take a preventive and proactive approach and encourage people with dementia, and those who support them, to be more active in ways that match their capabilities and interests. We need to encourage new initiatives that promote inclusion of people with dementia and that push the boundaries of our expectations to offer enjoyable, exciting pursuits for people with dementia.

Third, where the person with dementia has a family carer, that carer will influence the person's health and activity levels. We need to consider health and activity levels for both members of the couple together, their strengths and joint resources, and tailor services and support accordingly.

Reflections from the ALWAYs group

We thought that in order to promote physical activity for people with dementia and their carers, it would be useful to make a weekly list planning a few activities such as a walk around the block, finding a coffee shop if the area is not too rural, and so on. At the end of each day the person with dementia and their carer could tick off the achievements and carry others forward to the next day. The resulting sense of achievement could create a positive cycle where people with dementia increase their activity levels.

We discussed how carers and supporters, wanting to protect people with dementia, may unnecessarily limit physical activities rather than stretching their loved ones physically. Carers need to rethink which activities truly put people with dementia at risk of falls and injuries and encourage appropriate physical activity.

Key points

Key points for people with dementia and carers

- Stay as active as possible, as this will help maintain your well-being and protect you against other illnesses.
- Remind healthcare practitioners about all the health conditions you have.
- As a carer, by looking after your own health you are helping both yourself and the person you support.

Key points for health and social care practitioners

- Rather than just focusing on dementia, think about any other symptoms and health conditions that the person with dementia has.
- Ask people with dementia which health issues are having the greatest impact on their lives.
- Encourage people with dementia to engage in appropriate physical activity.

Key points for policy-makers

- Prioritise service models that are integrated and person-centred.
- Ensure the availability of suitable opportunities to exercise along with the necessary infrastructure.
- Promote awareness of the benefits of physical activity for people with dementia and carers.

 **Manifesto statement**

We want all our health needs to be treated in a way that fits with our requirements, regardless of age.

References

Alzheimer's Western Australia (n.d.) *Dementia and walking*. Available at: www.alzheimerswa.org.au/dementia-and-walking (accessed 5 September 2024).

Collins, R., Owen, S., Opdebeeck, C., et al. (2023) Provision of outdoor nature-based activity for older people with cognitive impairment: a scoping review from the ENLIVEN Project, *Health and Social Care in the Community*, 2023: 4574072. Available at: https://doi.org/10.1155/2023/4574072.

Delgado, J., Bowman, K. and Clare, L. (2020) Potentially inappropriate prescribing in dementia: a state-of-the-art review since 2007, *BMJ Open*, 10(1): e029172. Available at: https://doi.org/10.1136/bmjopen-2019-029172.

Evans, S. (2024) Connecting with nature, in K. Gray, C. Russell and J. Twigg (eds) *Leisure and Everyday Life with Dementia*. London: Open University Press.

Fielder, H. and Marsh, P. (2021) 'I used to be a gardener': connecting aged care residents to gardening and to each other through communal garden sites, *Australasian Journal on Ageing*, 40(1): e29–36.

Hillman, A., Rees Jones, I., Quinn, C., et al. (2023) The precariousness of living with, and caring for people with, dementia: insights from the IDEAL programme, *Social Science and Medicine*, 331: 116098. Available at: https://doi.org/10.1016/j.socscimed.2023.116098.

IDEAL Programme (2021) *Living with Dementia Toolkit*. Available at: https://livingwith-dementiatoolkit.org.uk/stay-active/ (accessed 5 September 2024).

Kitwood, T.M. (1997) *Dementia Reconsidered: The Person Comes First*, Buckingham: Open University Press.

Koch, T., Iliffe, S. and EVIDEM-ED project (2010) Rapid appraisal of barriers to the diagnosis and management of patients with dementia in primary care: a systematic review, *BMC Family Practice*, 11: 52. Available at: https://doi.org/10.1186/1471-2296-11-52.

Labirinto Cooperativa Sociale (n.d.) *Il Margherita inaugura il Giardino Alzheimer*. Available at: www.labirinto.coop/centro-margherita/giardino-alzheimer/ (accessed 5 September 2024).

Lutheran Community Services Northwest (n.d.) *Tacoma Zoo walk helps people with early stage memory loss*. Available at: www.lcsnw.org/2015/12/tacoma-zoo-walk-helps-people-with-early-stage-memory-loss (accessed 5 September 2024).

Nelis, S.M., Wu, Y.T., Matthews, F.E., et al. (2019) The impact of co-morbidity on the quality of life of people with dementia: findings from the IDEAL study, *Age and Ageing*, 48(3): 361–67.

Nuzum, H., Stickel, A., Corona, M., et al. (2020) Potential benefits of physical activity in MCI and dementia, *Behavioural Neurology*, 2020: 7807856. Available at: https://doi.org/10.1155/2020/7807856.

Opdebeeck, C., Katsaris, M.A., Martyr, A., et al. (2021) What are the benefits of pet ownership and care among people with mild-to-moderate dementia? Findings from the IDEAL programme, *Journal of Applied Gerontology*, 40(11): 1559–67.

Owen, S., Page, S.J., Ledingham, K., et al. (2024) Embodied leisure experiences of nature-based activities for people living with dementia, *Dementia*, 23(7): 1081–1102.

Page, S., Connell, J., Price, S., et al. (2023) Operationalizing transformative tourism: creating dementia-friendly outdoor and nature-based visitor experiences, *Journal of Travel Research*, 1(23). Available at: https://doi.org/10.1177/00472875231217735.

Poulos, C.J., Bayer, A., Beaupre, L., et al. (2017) A comprehensive approach to reablement in dementia, *Alzheimer's and Dementia: Translational Research and Clinical Interventions*, 3(3): 450–58.

Ramblers (n.d.) *Walking and dementia*. Available at: www.ramblers.org.uk/go-walking-hub/walking-and-dementia (accessed 5 September 2024).

Russell, C. (2024) Sport and physical activity, in K. Gray, C. Russell and J. Twigg (eds) *Leisure and Everyday Life with Dementia*. London: Open University Press.

Sabatini, S., Martyr, A., Hunt, A., et al. (2024) Comorbid health conditions and their impact on social isolation, loneliness, quality of life, and well-being in people with dementia: longitudinal findings from the IDEAL programme, *BMC Geriatrics*, 24: 23. Available at: https://doi.org/10.1186/s12877-023-04601-x.

Scottish Ballet (n.d.) *Time to Dance® On Demand: dementia-friendly resources to support brain health*. Available at: scottishballet.co.uk/move-with-us/dance-classes/time-to-dance/time-to-dance-on-demand/ (accessed 5 September 2024).

Sensory Trust (n.d.) *Activity groups*. Available at: www.sensorytrust.org.uk/projects/dementia/activity-groups (accessed 5 September 2024).

World Health Organization (WHO) (2020) *WHO guidelines on physical activity and sedentary behaviour*. Available at: https://www.who.int/publications/i/item/9789240015128.

Wu, Y.-T., Nelis, S.M., Quinn, C., et al. (2020) Factors associated with self- and informant ratings of quality of life, well-being and life satisfaction in people with mild-to-moderate dementia: results from the Improving the experience of Dementia and Enhancing Active Life programme, *Age and Ageing*, 49(3): 446–52.

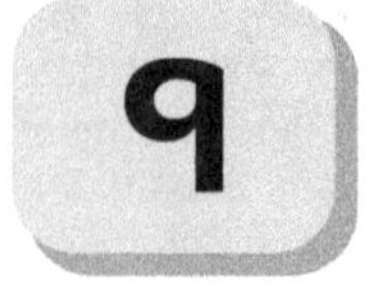

How you feel makes all the difference: psychological well-being

Linda Clare and Sally Stapley

(An IDEAL participant living with dementia)

In this chapter we will:

- explore what psychological well-being means when living with dementia
- explain why psychological well-being is crucial for people living with dementia
- consider what can help to improve psychological well-being

What do we mean by psychological well-being?

How we feel about ourselves and our lives is closely connected to whether we see ourselves as living well. In previous chapters, we have reflected on social resources, connections and relationships, physical fitness and health, and challenges in everyday life. All these domains contribute to how people feel. Psychological well-being is central to living well with dementia, and it is something we can influence and improve.

Psychological well-being reflects our personal, internal resources, built up over a lifetime of experiences. Kitwood described living with dementia as an interplay between neurological impairment, psychological resources, physical health, and social context (Kitwood, 1997). We have talked in previous chapters about how social resources and physical health help with living well. IDEAL evidence shows how, in the context of dementia-related changes in the brain, all these things influence psychological well-being.

The psychological resources that influence how people manage life with dementia include all the things that make up our sense of who we are:

- the dispositions, traits, and outlooks that form our personality
- the values, attitudes, and beliefs that shape how we think
- the emotional experiences that shape how we react and cope

Some of these are present throughout our lives, some evolve as we develop, and some change over time. Together they affect how we think and feel, and what we do. All this adds up to who we are, how we experience our sense of self, and how we evaluate our abilities.

Who we are – dispositions, traits, and outlooks

I think you've got to have a good outlook on life, because if you don't, you're not going to get any better, are you.
> (An IDEAL participant living with dementia)

Dispositions and traits are what we think of as forming our personality. Dispositions, such as whether we are excitable or more laid-back, are evident from birth, and contribute to the evolution of traits which are generally stable in adulthood. Researchers often think about these traits in terms of five dimensions:

- *Openness* – how open we are to new experiences
- *Conscientiousness* – how careful and disciplined we are
- *Extraversion* – how outgoing we are
- *Agreeableness* – how kind and considerate we are
- *Neuroticism* – how inclined we are to experience difficult emotions like fear, sadness, and anger

Where we sit on each of these five dimensions reflects our own unique personality profile. Traits are not easy to change, but over the course of our lives we can learn to work with the traits we have and build on our strengths. For example, people who are not very outgoing and need time alone, described as introverts, will prefer interactions with one or a few people to the kinds of large group activities that more outgoing extraverts thrive on. People can learn to choose the kinds of situations where they are comfortable. Traits are neither good nor bad in themselves, and the same characteristic can be helpful in some circumstances and not others. For example, being disciplined with pursuing challenging goals can pay off for young people but may be less helpful later in life, when the ability to flexibly adapt can be more beneficial.

Dispositions and traits combine with experience to shape people's outlook on themselves, the world, and the future. This is reflected in psychological resources such as:

- *Self-esteem* – how people evaluate their own worth
- *Self-efficacy* – the extent to which people feel in control and able to manage
- *Optimism* – hope about the future and expectation of positive outcomes in the face of adversity

It is easy to see how developing dementia could challenge a person's sense of self-worth, self-efficacy, and optimism.

IDEAL participants were like any group of adults in that scores on the five personality dimensions stayed the same over time (Hunt et al., 2023). In general, personality does not change as a person develops dementia, but dementia can make it harder to manage in ways that suit a person's characteristics. While traits are mostly stable, dementia-related changes in the brain can sometimes affect the expression of these traits so that personality appears to change. This can be distressing especially for family carers. People who scored higher for openness, conscientiousness, agreeableness, and extraversion tended to have better scores for living well, but people who were more prone to experiencing difficult emotions tended to have lower scores for living well (Hunt et al., 2023). People who had a stronger sense of self-worth, felt more in control, and were more optimistic were more likely to see themselves as living well (Lamont et al., 2020).

We need to take account of different dispositions and traits when planning support, and make sure there are options to suit different preferences. We need to know more about how to support people who experience difficult emotions and how to help people maintain, regain, or improve their sense of self-worth, control, and optimism. We need better evidence about the kinds of talking and other non-drug treatments that are helpful for people with dementia. Alongside this, encouraging peer support, adapting environments and contexts, and sharing strategies to make it easier for people to manage independently and keep doing the things they enjoy are crucial.

How we think – values, attitudes, and beliefs

I think it's how I do it, you know. I make it good or bad.
(An IDEAL participant living with dementia)

The values people hold, and their attitudes and beliefs, affect how they react to developing and living with dementia, as we saw in Chapter 2. For example, people who think of it as a disease score lower for quality of life than those who see it as part of ageing, while people who believe in managing independently without professional help may be reluctant to seek a dementia diagnosis. Here, we will think about two other aspects of values, attitudes, and beliefs: ageing and religion/spirituality.

In the IDEAL cohort, more than one in three were aged 80 or above, and more than nine out of ten were aged over 65. Over our lifetimes, we develop a set of beliefs about ageing in general and our own future ageing. Realistically, ageing presents challenges and comes with greater likelihood of health problems, but often attitudes are shaped by negative stereotypes and expectations and can be unduly pessimistic. People with dementia who approached getting older with more positive attitudes, or who said they felt younger than their actual age, had better scores for living well and were less likely to feel depressed (Sabatini et al., 2021).

We thought that religious practice or spiritual beliefs might better enable people to cope with dementia. More than nine out of ten cohort participants said they identified with a religion, a much higher proportion than in the wider UK population, but less than half said they prayed or went to religious services. Fewer than two-thirds said that spirituality was important to them. We found no links between religious practice or spiritual beliefs and capability to live well.

How we feel – emotional states

It saddens me a bit really that I realise I am not as mentally astute as I used to be.

(An IDEAL participant living with dementia)

Dispositions, traits, and outlooks shape our emotional experience. People who are worriers or tend to ruminate will be more likely to feel anxious or depressed, and people who feel in control and hopeful about the future will be more likely to feel content. Adverse circumstances can tip us into distressing emotional states. How we are and how we think influences our ability to cope with adversity. It can be hard to manage difficult emotions, but unlike traits, states are changeable. Sometimes depression and anxiety can be with us for a while but then improve. At other times, people may need help and support to overcome these difficulties. A complication for people with dementia is that changes in the brain resulting from the condition can also directly affect emotional state. It can be hard to distinguish what is due to brain changes and what is due to circumstances, and how these different aspects affect coping.

Researchers have described two main ways in which people cope with challenges. Generally, people use both but are more inclined to adopt one rather than the other. One involves focusing on managing emotions. Faced with a situation that arouses anxiety, a person who tends to cope in this emotion-focused way will try to reduce anxiety and may avoid the situation altogether, which could be counter-productive. The other involves focusing on problem-solving.

A person who tends to cope in this way might look for ways to manage the situation, for example finding out more about what is involved or planning ahead. People who coped by trying to solve problems tended to have better living well scores than people who coped by focusing on their emotions (Clare et al., 2022).

Between one-quarter and one-third of the IDEAL cohort had scores indicating they were depressed, although these were not necessarily the same people at each time point. Not surprisingly, people experiencing depression were less likely to feel they were living well (Wu et al., 2021). However, IDEAL has also shown how resilient many people with dementia can be. This was especially striking in how they coped with the COVID-19 pandemic. The pandemic did have an impact on how people felt; living with social restrictions was challenging, and people on average felt lonelier and a little less satisfied with their lives. Notably, though, during the pandemic, people with dementia were less likely to feel depressed or pessimistic, and their ratings of well-being and quality of life were the same as before the pandemic (Sabatini et al., 2022).

Supporting people to manage transient negative emotional states and providing more in-depth help where these persist is important. This could be through talking therapies or other non-drug treatments, building coping skills, or offering activities that help people focus on their strengths. Evidence about how best to do this is limited (NICE, 2018) and people with dementia have little access to these kinds of treatments. However, a growing understanding of how we can help people with dementia to talk about what is happening to them is explored in another book in this series (Cheston, 2022).

Alongside this, changes in people's environment and situation could help. About one in three people with dementia in the IDEAL cohort felt lonely, so reducing feelings of loneliness, such as through peer support, could be a powerful way of improving emotional state. Depression is not just a matter for the individual. If a person with dementia who has a family carer is experiencing depression, it is likely that the carer will be affected too, and vice versa (Wu et al., 2021). The positive aspect of this is that helping one member of the couple with depression should also be helpful for the other.

How we act – what we do and why

While you're busy and you get on with people, you're enjoying life.
(An IDEAL participant living with dementia)

Doing activities we enjoy, whatever they are, is important for well-being. Keeping occupied gives us enjoyment and a sense of purpose, with group activities providing opportunities to socialise and meet new people. Our interests are also part of who we are; for example, the retired cook who still likes to bake, or the lifelong sports enthusiast who wants to find an accessible sport in older age.

In our conversational interviews with IDEAL participants, one person we spoke to had problems with her memory and finding words but working on her allotment had helped her to focus on what she could still do: '*When I'm doing things, I can forget that I haven't got a good memory because it doesn't matter anymore*'. Continuing interests or hobbies can help emphasise the person's abilities and help them to feel happier. Missing out on doing purposeful things can be difficult: '*if I can keep my mind going and keep busy, I'm alright. Once I lose them things, I get so miserable*'. Doing activities with other people is an important way of making new friends and getting social support, such as at a singing group or dementia café: '*it's the company, everybody in the same boat, all rowing together, and that makes a world of difference to me*'.

Some people might give up an interest or lose enjoyment because they doubt their abilities, lack self-confidence, or compare their current skills negatively with past proficiencies; examples include an artist who had avoided painting for three years and a craftsman who had left his new printing press untouched. Giving up interests can affect psychological well-being, especially when associated with loss of skills or even loss of identity. Encouraging the person to resume previous interests may be possible with appropriate support, or it might be possible to develop a new interest. The important point is to find something you enjoy doing: '*I don't think it matters what the activity is ... anything. Everybody can find a hobby ... You must challenge yourself. Every day, you've got to get up and think, what can I do?*' Keeping the brain active through hobbies or even just maintaining the daily routine was important for our interviewees.

Using time meaningfully and doing activities we enjoy is essential for psychological well-being. However, where people are managing other health conditions, there is a risk that the importance of occupation is overlooked in favour of meeting physical care needs (Hansen et al., 2017). Professionals need to be aware of how important pursuing activities and interests is for living well. They have an important role to play in enabling people with dementia to engage in activities they enjoy. Remaining cognisant of the importance of pursuing activities and interests for living well can inform both occupational therapy and psychological support. A more detailed discussion of everyday and leisure activities is presented in another book in this series (Gray et al., 2024).

How we see ourselves – self-concept

I don't get really upset because I think to myself, don't be so stupid ... but yes, I can cry, I've never been a crying person, even when I was normal as I put it.
(An IDEAL participant living with dementia)

We go through life feeling that we are the same person, even though we change over time. Typically, people have a coherent sense of who they are in the here-and-now that reaches back into the past and forward into the future. This stable sense of self is entirely personal, and although we can try to describe it, no-one else can see it or measure it. Alongside this, we know many things about ourselves – what kind of person we are, what we believe, what has happened to us – and this accumulated knowledge forms our mental picture of who we are, our self-concept. This is more visible to others and can be shared and even measured.

We know from people living with mild-to-moderate dementia that their self-concept stays with them, even if they forget some specific information about themselves (Caddell and Clare, 2010). However, sometimes things happen that disrupt the continuity of our sense of self and make us feel we are not the 'same person' anymore. Dementia can be one of those things. In the IDEAL cohort, one in five of the participants with dementia said they no longer felt they were the same person they had always been (Clare et al., 2020). These people had poorer psychological well-being, scored lower for self-esteem, self-efficacy, attitudes to their own ageing, mood, and optimism, were lonelier, and had poorer scores for living well. If people say they no longer feel they are the same person, this could be a signal that they need psychological support. Talking to people sensitively to explore what this means to them could help to identify what kind of support would be useful. Focusing on what people know about themselves could help to reconnect people with the feeling of being the same person and reduce psychological discomfort.

How we appraise our abilities – awareness

I used to cook quite a lot ... I can't risk that, because with hot stuff around I can drop it and I mean accidentally ... I'm afraid of trying it ... I don't want to hurt myself or my wife.

(An IDEAL participant living with dementia)

We all vary in how accurately we appraise our own abilities and performance. Our self-knowledge includes many appraisals of this kind – whether we are good at sport, whether we have a good memory, and so on. Sometimes we overestimate; surveys show that about 80 per cent of people consider their driving ability to be above average, although this is a mathematical impossibility. Sometimes we underestimate, for example if we feel low or depressed, or lacking in self-esteem and confidence. Our judgements are not necessarily just a product of our own psychological resources. Feedback from others can help us adjust our own evaluations but might be ignored if it seems too different to how we perceive ourselves. Sometimes we decide to present ourselves in particular ways, either consciously or without really being aware of it. For example, we might want to seem more confident and able than we really are when being interviewed for an exciting job.

Some kinds of brain injury can affect this process of appraisal, sometimes to the extent that people lack awareness and cannot realistically appraise their performance or grasp what has happened to them. Unfortunately, it is still often said that people with dementia lack awareness, lack insight, or display anosognosia – a Greek word meaning 'without knowledge of disease' used to refer to unawareness or denial of a disease or neurological impairment. In dementia, changes in the brain are more subtle than in sudden major brain injury, although they still have an impact on awareness (Clare et al., 2012). Most people with mild-to-moderate dementia have some awareness of the difficulties posed by their dementia, although making accurate appraisals may be challenging. Only a few people in the IDEAL cohort, 7 out of 100, said they had no dementia-related difficulties at all (Clare et al., 2022). A larger proportion, about 11 in every 100, had exceptionally high awareness of difficulties, while for the rest awareness was reasonably aligned to actual abilities (Alexander et al., 2021). Lack of awareness is often spoken of as fixed and lasting, but it can be transient. Most of the people who said they had no dementia-related difficulties at the outset acknowledged some difficulties one or two years later. It could be that as their dementia progressed, difficulties became more obvious, or they adjusted to living with the condition. Only five of the people we were able to follow up continued to say they had none of the common difficulties associated with dementia throughout a two-year period (Alexander et al., 2022).

Awareness is important because it affects how people with dementia manage living with the condition and how they interact with others:

- Difficulty judging how one is doing while engaging in specific activities could lead to problems and mean people are less safe.
- Difficulty evaluating how capable one is in various activities could create difficulties with planning or making decisions.
- Difficulty grasping the wider implications of having dementia might make planning for the future or deciding how to manage other health problems more challenging.

While more awareness can be helpful, it does have a downside. People in the IDEAL cohort who were more aware about their dementia-related difficulties had lower scores for living well and more signs of depression (Alexander et al., 2021).

Understanding a person's awareness is central to understanding what kinds of support will be beneficial. In some situations, it could be helpful to take a formal look at a person's awareness. Awareness is complex and involves making judgements about different kinds of things. A person might make accurate appraisals in one area but less so in another. The kinds of detailed questionnaires employed in research about awareness are too long and complicated for everyday use (Clare et al., 2011). Building on what we learned about awareness in IDEAL, we developed the Health Awareness Profile Interview (HAPI), a 10-minute structured interview that can be done in person or by telephone or videoconference (Alexander et al., 2024). The HAPI explores awareness in the domains of dementia-related difficulties, memory and functional ability, medication management (where relevant), relationships, and mobility. Health and care practitioners can use the HAPI when taking a formal look at someone's awareness.

So what does this tell us about reconsidering living with dementia?

We began by saying that psychological well-being is something we can potentially influence and improve. Previous chapters have pointed to the importance of creating communities, environments, and contexts that can support and enhance psychological well-being. The more individual focus of this chapter emphasises that to maintain or improve psychological well-being, it is crucial to understand each person, focus on strengths, and personalise support. This does not necessarily require specialist knowledge but rather sensitivity, imagination, and flexibility. Where challenges to psychological well-being are significant and long-lasting, however, there is an urgent need for evidence about what kinds of talking and other non-drug treatments are helpful and for effective evidence-based treatments to be made accessible. Promoting psychological well-being should be at the heart of our endeavours.

Reflections from the ALWAYs group

This chapter has some important messages for practitioners. It is vital to think about us as people, and not just in terms of dementia. We want you to find out about the lives we have lived and what we are like as individuals, because this will help you connect us with the kinds of activities and people that can improve our well-being. We want you to be sensitive to what we need, and to our worries and fears. Please ask us how we are and how we feel, and make sure anyone who needs more help with mood or with adjusting to the changes dementia brings can get it.

We also reflected on how carers are key to supporting well-being and how carers themselves need support to do this – whether that is encouragement to allow for a degree of risk, or acknowledgement of how hard it is to see the person with dementia changing.

Key points

Key points for people with dementia and carers

- Depression and anxiety are common but often improve with time.
- Seek help if these or other distressing emotions are severe and persistent.
- Try to focus on strengths and stay connected with the things that define who you are.

Key points for health and social care professionals

- Take time to understand the person with dementia.
- Explore how the person feels but do so sensitively.
- Think creatively about how to support or improve the person's psychological well-being.

Key points for policy-makers

- Understand that support for people with dementia must be tailored to individual needs.
- Consider how services can offer personalised support.
- Develop the evidence base on effective non-drug treatments that address challenges to psychological well-being.

 **Manifesto statement**

We want our well-being to be supported and to be seen for who we really are.

References

Alexander, C.M., Martyr, A., Gamble, L.D., et al. (2021) Does awareness of condition help people with mild-to-moderate dementia to live well? Findings from the IDEAL programme, *BMC Geriatrics*, 21: 511. Available at: https://doi.org/10.1186/s12877-021-02468-4.

Alexander, C.M., Martyr, A. and Clare, L. (2022) Changes in awareness of condition in people with mild-to-moderate dementia: longitudinal findings from the IDEAL cohort, *International Journal of Geriatric Psychiatry*, 37(4): e5702. Available at: https://doi.org/10.1002/gps.5702.

Alexander, C.M., Martyr, A. and Clare, L. (2024) The Healthcare Awareness Profile Interview: development of a new evidence-based brief clinical tool to assess awareness in people with dementia, *Neuropsychological Rehabilitation*. Available at: https://doi.org/10.1080/09602011.2024.2337152.

Caddell, L.S. and Clare, L. (2010) The impact of dementia on self and identity: a systematic review, *Clinical Psychology Review*, 30(1): 113–26.

Cheston, R. (2022) *Dementia and Psychotherapy Reconsidered.* London: Open University Press.

Clare, L., Whitaker, C.J., Nelis, S.M., et al. (2011) Multidimensional assessment of awareness in early-stage dementia: a cluster analytic approach, *Dementia and Geriatric Cognitive Disorders*, 31(5): 317–27.

Clare, L., Nelis, S.M., Martyr, A., et al. (2012) The influence of psychological, social and contextual factors on the expression and measurement of awareness in early-stage dementia: testing a biopsychosocial model, *International Journal of Geriatric Psychiatry*, 27(2): 167–77.

Clare, L., Martyr, A., Morris, R.G., et al. (2020) Discontinuity in the subjective experience of self among people with mild-to-moderate dementia is associated with poorer psychological health: findings from the IDEAL cohort, *Journal of Alzheimer's Disease*, 77(1): 127–38.

Clare, L., Gamble, L.D., Martyr, A., et al. (2022) Psychological processes in adapting to dementia: illness representations among the IDEAL cohort, *Psychology and Aging*, 37(4): 524–41.

Gray, K., Russell, C. and Twigg, J. (eds) (2024) *Leisure and Everyday Life with Dementia*. London: Open University Press.

Hansen, A., Hauge, S. and Bergland, Å. (2017) Meeting psychosocial needs for persons with dementia in home care services: a qualitative study of different perceptions and practices among health care providers, *BMC Geriatrics*, 17: 211. Available at: https://doi.org/10.1186/s12877-017-0612-3.

Hunt, A., Martyr, A., Gamble, L.D., et al. (2023) The associations between personality traits and quality of life, satisfaction with life, and well-being over time in people with dementia and their caregivers: findings from the IDEAL programme, *BMC Geriatrics*, 23: 354. Available at: https://doi.org/10.1186/s12877-023-04075-x.

Kitwood, T. (1997) *Dementia Reconsidered: The Person Comes First*. Buckingham: Open University Press.

Lamont, R.A., Nelis, S.M., Quinn, C., et al. (2020) Psychological predictors of 'living well' with dementia: findings from the IDEAL study, *Aging and Mental Health*, 24(6): 956–64.

National Institute for Health and Care Excellence (NICE) (2018) *Dementia: assessment, management and support for people living with dementia and their carers*, NICE Guideline NG97. Available at: https://www.nice.org.uk/guidance/ng97 (accessed 10 September 2024).

Sabatini, S., Ukoumunne, O.C., Martyr, A., et al. (2021) Relationship between self-perceptions of aging and 'living well' among people with mild-to-moderate dementia: findings from the IDEAL Programme, *Archives of Gerontology and Geriatrics*, 94: 104328. Available at: https://doi.org/10.1016/j.archger.2020.104328.

Sabatini, S., Bennett, H.Q., Martyr, A., et al. (2022) Minimal impact of COVID-19 on the mental health and well-being of people living with dementia: analysis on matched longitudinal data from the IDEAL study. *Frontiers in Psychiatry*, 13: 849808. Available at: https://doi.org/10.3389/fpsyt.2022.849808.

Wu, Y.-T., Clare, L. and Matthews, F.E. (2021) Relationship between depressive symptoms and capability to live well in people with dementia and their carers: results from the Improving the experience of Dementia and Enhancing Active Life (IDEAL) programme, *Aging and Mental Health*, 25(1): 38–45.

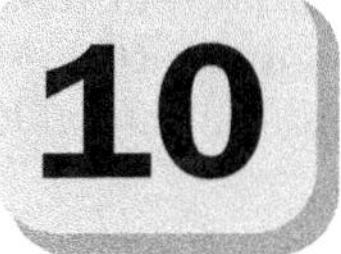

Is there anybody out there? Services and support

Catherine Charlwood and Hayley Hogan

There's a lot out there but I just need to ask, and there's a barrier I feel to being able to ask.

(Quinn et al., 2022b: 848)

In this chapter we will:

- think about the types of services and support which improve life with dementia
- consider patterns of service use and how much these cost
- question why access to, and experiences of, services and support vary

Health and humanity

This book demonstrates how many aspects of life contribute to the experience of living with dementia. We have heard about social connections, everyday activities, psychological well-being, and physical health.

IDEAL has always sought to exemplify that health can only be authentically understood by looking at this broader picture. This aligns with new understandings from the World Health Organization (WHO), who have acknowledged 'human functioning' as a central concept. If we measure population health, we might know about the prevalence of disease, but not how people feel about their lives or how they live them. Age and life are very different things, for both the individual and society. Human functioning considers not just biological health – what we might call physical health – but also lived health. Lived health includes 'the actual performance of activities in the physical, human-built, attitudinal, and social environments that constitute the person's complete lived context' (Bickenbach et al., 2023: 4). This mirrors how IDEAL has studied dementia, in the context of people's real-life experiences. For instance, when we asked people with dementia and carers what could be changed in the local community to enable people to live well with dementia, people spoke not just about increased awareness and understanding of dementia, but also the need for dementia-friendly signage, more benches, better transport, and well-maintained footpaths, acknowledging both the physical and human-built environment (Quinn et al., 2022a).

The concept of human functioning helps us consider the topic of services and support by keeping in view the ways in which the experience of living with dementia might benefit from support. Here, we consider what IDEAL reveals about the services and support people with dementia and carers access (or wish to), the relative cost of different types of service and support, and barriers to accessing them. Throughout, there is an emphasis on the need for a variety of options to suit different needs and preferences, to focus on what matters to the person and their network. We will call this 'personalised support'.

The full spectrum of services and support

Dementia itself is a complex jigsaw of experiences. Accessing services and support is another jigsaw entirely, one where people may feel they have no guiding picture to follow. If we want to reconsider living with dementia, then we need to look at how an overarching offer of services and support could be made accessible to those who need it.

Fragmentation of services and support leaves people unsure of what is available, or who is responsible for which part:

> Dementia is a complex condition crossing primary, secondary, community, acute and social care. This complexity inevitably leads to a lack of ownership of the condition within the health and care system, which creates variation in the quality and type of support people receive.
>
> (Alzheimer's Society, 2022: 4)

While dementia is a useful case study in complexity, part of the reason for thinking in terms of functioning is because 'the political, administrative, and policy bifurcation between "health" and "social" hampers policy action to improve population health' (Bickenbach et al., 2023: 7). This demonstrates unhelpful divisions within the landscape of services and support.

To provide clarity in what follows, we separate health and social care provision. However, these divisions are rarely clear-cut. While the exact role names and divisions of services differ between countries, the split between health services and social care services (structurally and financially) is largely universal. Our discussion of services will be based on the UK context, as this is the context in which IDEAL was conducted. In the UK, the NHS provides universal healthcare free at the point of delivery, but social care often incurs a cost to the individual or family. We acknowledge that although many components will be similar across countries, the exact mix and the costs to individuals will vary.

There are multiple reasons why people with dementia need to engage with health services, summarised in Figure 10.1, and many of the professionals and

Figure 10.1: Possible reasons for interactions with health services.

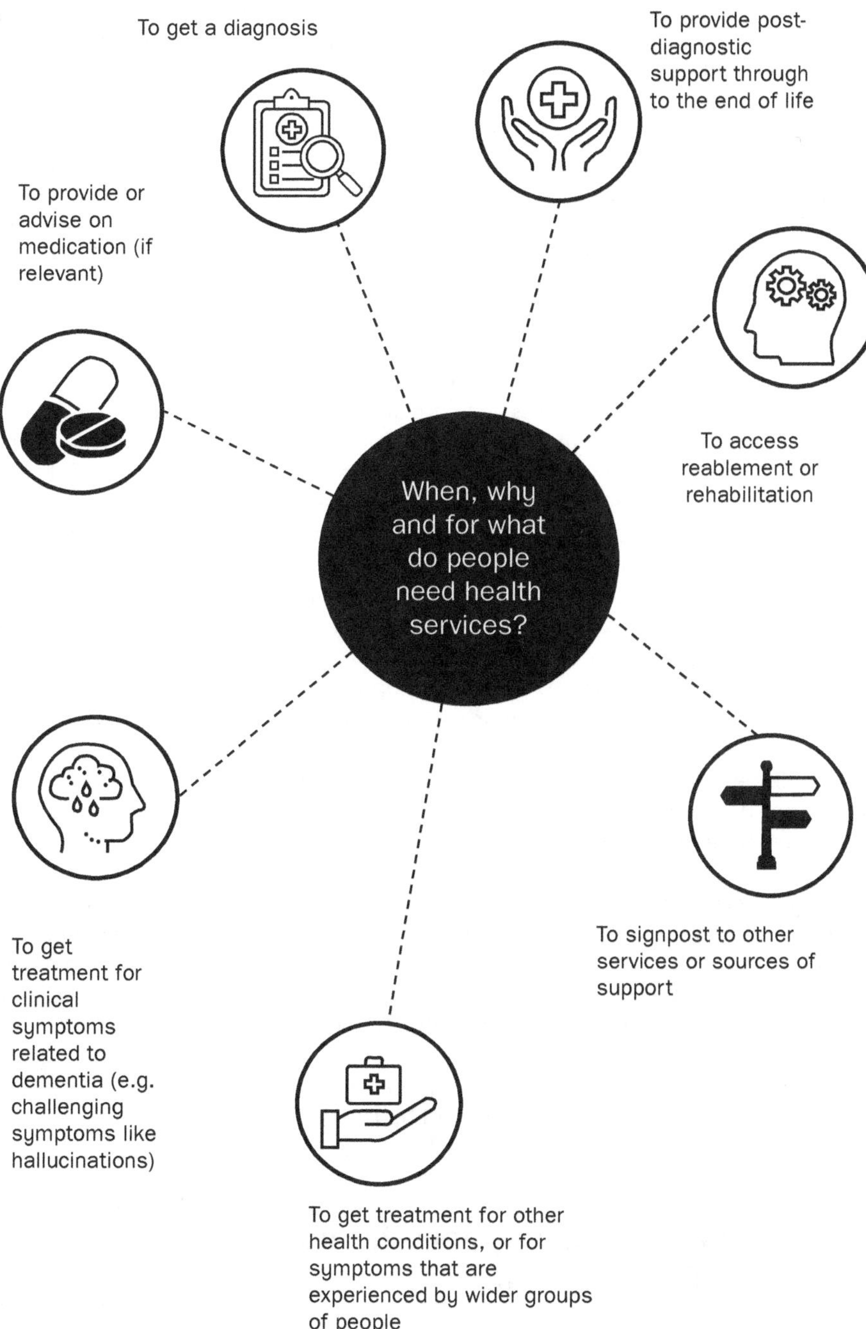

practitioners who people affected by dementia might meet are not dementia specialists. General practitioners have expressed low confidence in providing care for patients with dementia, particularly in the post-diagnostic stage (Tang et al., 2018). As Chapter 8 showed, we need to look at health holistically so that practitioners can respond helpfully: they may need some dementia training. The ALWAYs group highlighted this through the example of seeking support from an incontinence nurse. In one case, access to products was through a confusing set of questions over the phone and then a request for more was met with derision. In another, a mountain of sanitary products turned up on the doorstep, but the person had forgotten the conversation. The ALWAYs group agreed that no-one should feel, or be made to feel, embarrassed about incontinence. Resolving incontinence issues can enable a person with dementia and the person supporting them to feel more confident going out.

Social care services comprise local authority teams, including social workers and occupational therapists, private in-home care providers, voluntary sector provision in the community such as day centres, activity groups, dementia cafés and meeting centres, and care homes or nursing homes, which are usually privately run (see Figure 10.2). Social care services tend to come with a cost in the UK, although Scotland provides some free personal care for adults.

Beyond health and social care services, there is a whole range of support provided by the voluntary sector, community groups, and more (see Figure 10.3).

Support can also be a lot closer to home. People with dementia need the support of their family and friends. Social support and stimulation are crucial to quality of life. Sadly, however, many people say that they lose friends after being diagnosed. *'The younger men in my family don't know how to behave around me and so find it easier not to see me'*, one woman told us. While support could be a six-week course, support can also be social and simple. Chris, a member of the ALWAYs group, who lives with frontotemporal dementia and is a keen brass band member, gave this example:

> *The guy that sits next to me is very helpful in subtle ways. If we're told to go from a certain place on the piece of music, because I've lost my alphabet now and my numbers, I can't. He will lean forward and he'll count on his own music which bar it's going to be, as if he needs to know … It just gives you a little bit of a warm tingle, that you know somebody's got your back.*

Having outlined what may be available, we turn to what we discovered about the services and support accessed by the IDEAL cohort.

Which services and support did people use and what did they cost?

There are national recommendations about the type of services and support that people living with dementia and carers should receive (NICE, 2018).

Figure 10.2: Possible reasons for involvement of social care services.

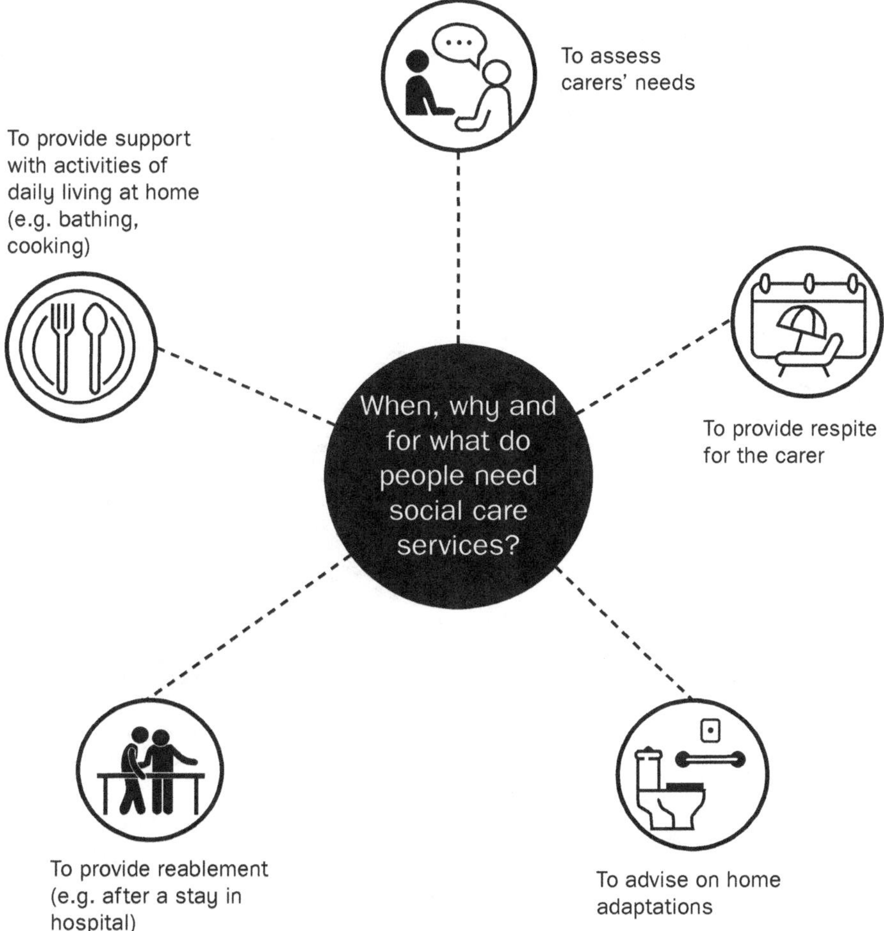

Everybody should receive this support, but only half the people IDEAL asked said they had. This is within a UK context, but the issues may be relevant more widely. Age, gender, and educational level all appeared to make a difference in how much support people received. We found that older women with lower levels of education got less support. The relationship between the person with dementia and the carer also made a difference: if they were married or partners, both received less support. However, people with dementia supported by a spouse or partner attended more psychosocial interventions, 'reiterating the important role carers may play in facilitating the use of support services' (van Horik et al., 2022: 6). The questions did not uncover the reasons why people were accessing services (or not), only whether they were. We look at external barriers to access later.

Figure 10.3: Possible reasons for interactions with voluntary sector or community services.

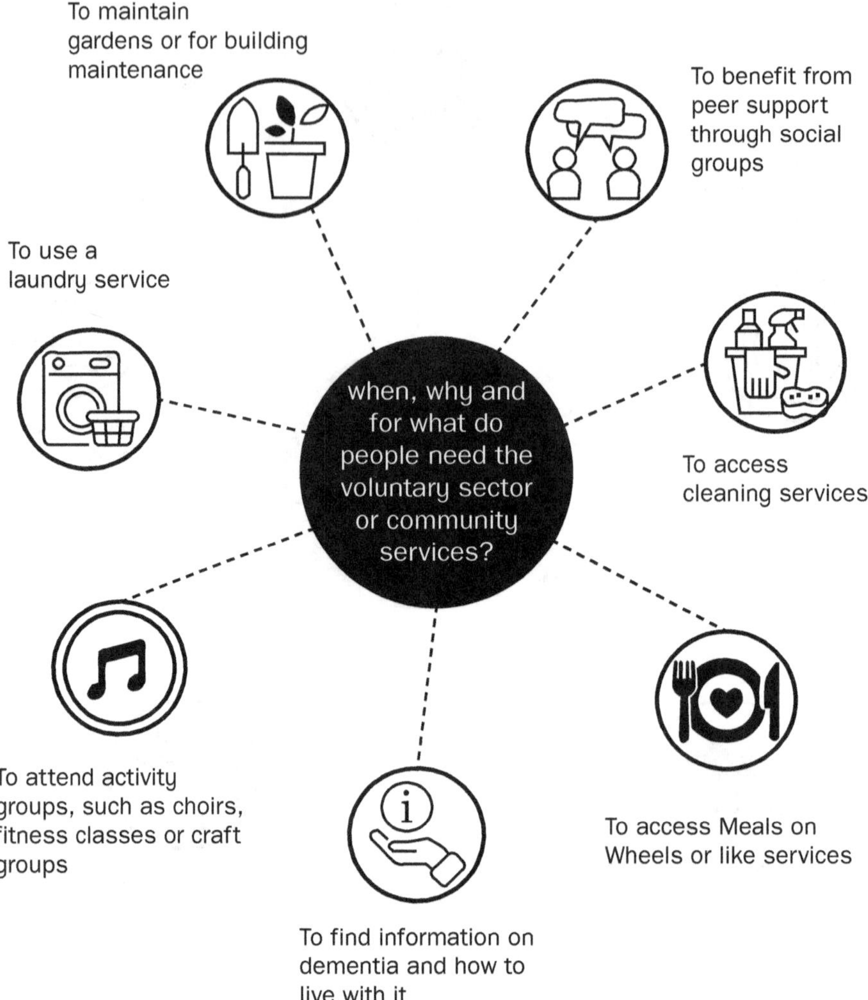

We also wanted to understand how much services and support cost, and how costs change over time. This is, of course, limited to our cohort of people living with mild-to-moderate dementia and their carers in the community. We only know about people who stayed in the cohort; people who moved into residential care would incur increased costs. However, the data reveal some important patterns (see Figure 10.4).

When we added up the costs of all health and social care service use, out-of-pocket payments for things like home equipment or a cleaner, and unpaid care by costing hours spent caring at the national minimum wage, the picture

Figure 10.4: Mean costs of services and support for IDEAL participants over a three-month period.

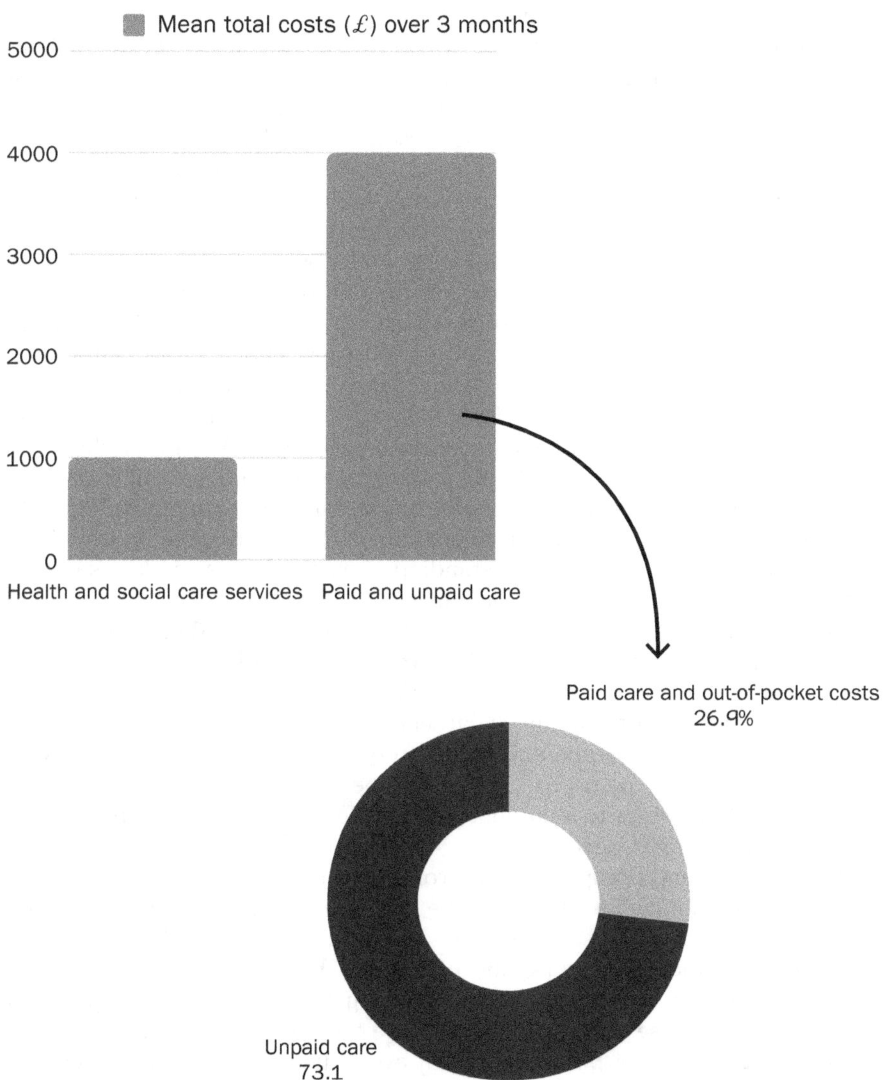

was stark. Three-quarters of the total costs for this group were accounted for by unpaid care (Henderson et al., 2019). Over time, although use and cost of services went up, the amount and cost of carers' time also increased. As seen in Chapter 2, people have differing support needs and society needs to acknowledge and meet these requirements.

How could we better support individuals through the complex services system, given that dementia is unpredictable and needs change over time? A key issue for IDEAL was understanding whether people have access to a named professional. In the UK, it is recommended that each person living with dementia be provided 'with a single named health or social care professional who is responsible for coordinating their care' (NICE, 2018: 19). The professional should act as a named point of contact who you can email or call any time for advice. However, only about one-third of the IDEAL cohort had a named professional and for some of them this person was in place because of another condition; for example, it could be a specialist diabetes or Parkinson's disease nurse. Few people with dementia currently have access to a named professional in the form of a dementia support worker.

A named professional of this kind helps with continuity of care and understanding the individual situation. During the COVID-19 pandemic, people felt that 'if the practitioner did not know them, any changes in their dementia-related needs would not be understood' (Pentecost et al., 2022). One person sought to be proactive about their decline and went to see the doctor but found that *references I made to how I thought things had changed were dismissed in saying, "Well, you know, dementia does progress"*. A general statement about dementia applied to an individual situation can be not just unhelpful, but hurtful, and possibly prevent someone from seeking future support. While the doctor correctly notes that dementia progresses, having a named professional enables a more personalised understanding of what progression looks like for that individual and strategies to manage it.

A dementia support worker can act as the nominated lead professional following diagnosis, ensuring a smoother transition from specialist care to the complex post-diagnostic services landscape. Dementia support workers have knowledge of a range of available local services, providing advice and information for people with dementia and their carers, including accessing wider care and support services as needs change and become more complex (Goeman et al., 2016). Better links to a navigator-type role can also address information and social engagement needs.

However, dementia support worker roles need to be properly resourced and staff given a manageable caseload. The ALWAYs group also highlighted how many different names these roles take: dementia navigators/advisers/support workers/link workers/referrers, and community-based roles such as village/community agents. Not everyone can identify the support that might exist in their area, because they do not recognise the name. These inconsistences exacerbate the so-called 'postcode lottery' even when services exist; where you happen to live may grant or deny you access to support.

Our research during the COVID-19 pandemic taught us useful lessons. While some people with dementia preferred face-to-face medical appointments, others found online or telephone appointments convenient for certain purposes. Many people spoke about how much they valued 'check-in' or welfare calls from services. This offers a solution for ongoing provision: where people have difficulty accessing services, through living in rural areas or being unable to drive, services could reach out in this low-cost way.

Supporting the supporter: How do services serve carers?

Most of the support for people with dementia in the IDEAL cohort came from unpaid carers. Family members and friends provide support for people with dementia, but they themselves also need support. This could be advice, help navigating the benefits system, peer support from other carers, or having their own needs assessed, which is an entitlement in the UK.

Dementia presents a steep learning curve for the carer. Many people only learn about dementia as it enters their life. At Time 1, 72 per cent of carers had received information or educational materials about dementia (see Figure 10.5).

Figure 10.5: An overview of carer access to information at Time 1 (T1) of IDEAL.

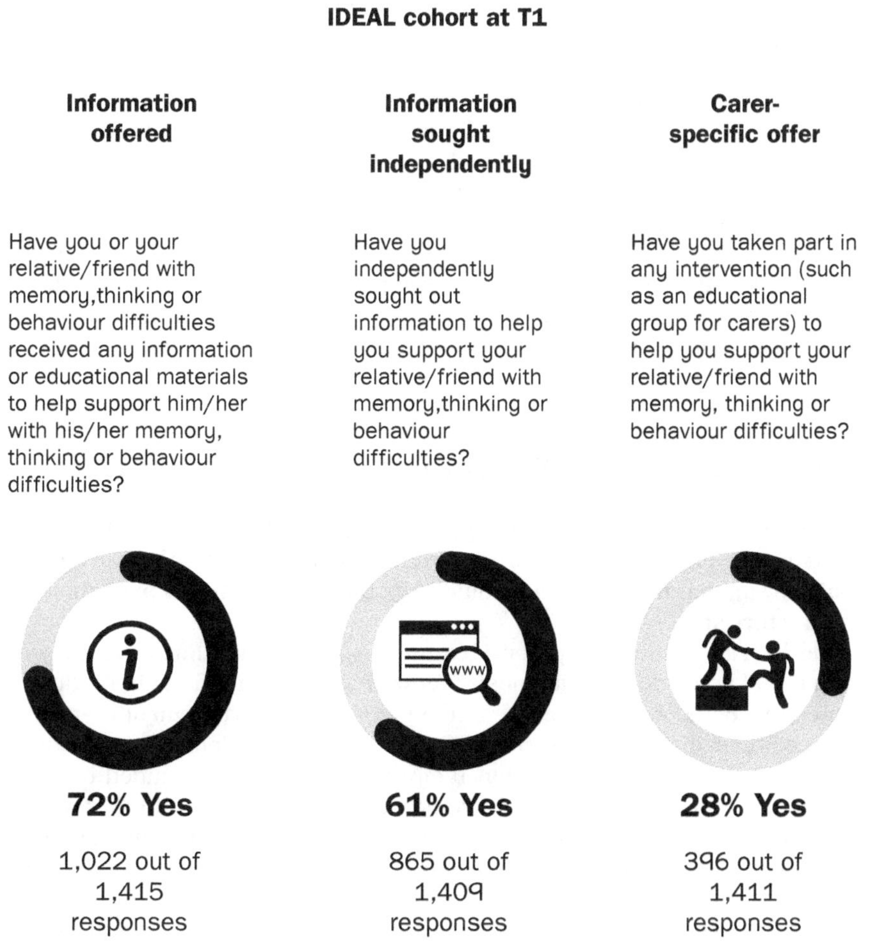

IDEAL cohort at T1

The caveat was that this information could be for either the carer or the person with dementia. Few had received carer-specific help despite the fact that offering 'carers of people living with dementia a psychoeducation and skills training intervention' is recommended (NICE, 2018: 33).

Supporting carers is important, not just for their own well-being, but also for the well-being of the person with dementia. As we saw in Chapter 6, dyadic influences have a big impact. It is vital that carers are supported both emotionally and practically to reduce stress levels and increase feelings of competence, and that they are able to access help when needed (Quinn et al., 2020). As Figure 10.5 shows, 61 per cent of carers independently sought information about dementia. While many sourced this from charities like Alzheimer's Society and Dementia UK, 'Google' or 'the internet' were cited by many people, leaving them at risk of potentially accessing misinformation. It further suggests that carers are heavily reliant on their own energies and digital know-how to find information.

We must also remember that many carers can be older and have health conditions of their own. Some were accessing online information by proxy, *'from my daughter who searches the internet'*, with a lucky few able to access local groups. While it is heartening to know that carers are seeking information, this puts carer support on shaky ground; a dementia diagnosis is a time of upheaval, and external direction from those with knowledge of dementia would free carers up to devote time to their own well-being, rather than needing to search for information.

Carer groups, where people want them, are an important source of support. Being able to speak to others in the same situation can help people to feel less alone, to problem-solve, and to reduce feelings of guilt. Groups may meet in-person or online and can provide an important release valve.

What prevents people from accessing services?

While financial resources remain a problem worldwide and demand continues to outstrip supply, we can think about what could be done at little or low cost. It is easy to say that more funding would help, but this does not explain the many other factors at work.

One barrier to accessing services and support is readiness: is someone ready to acknowledge the diagnosis? As well as being emotionally ready, people need to be cognitively ready. Some people who have dementia are more aware of their diagnosis and the difficulties of having dementia than others (see Chapter 9). When asked what they thought could be changed to enable people with dementia to live well, some people said things like *'Not sure as these are early days'*. It is important to recognise that people may need different types of support as they become more aware of difficulties with dementia: the right support, at the right time.

A diagnosis is usually what grants access to dementia services and support. However, not everyone wishes to seek a diagnosis, sometimes due to previous bad experiences. While people were quick to acknowledge that services were often under-resourced and staffed by well-meaning individuals, we also heard comments like this: *'You've got to get to rock bottom before anybody will help you. Shout, scream, and even that's not enough sometimes … they don't tell you where the help is either'* (Henley et al., 2023: 2055). Given this type of experience, some people will understandably not seek help. There is a global drive to increase diagnosis rates, but this needs to be followed by appropriate and meaningful post-diagnostic support.

Once people have a diagnosis these inequalities in access to, and experiences of, services and support continue. We can think about why in terms of suitability, accessibility, and availability. Suitability determines whether someone makes use of available services. There are many reasons why people might find services unsuitable. When we spoke with community leaders of people from South Asian or Caribbean backgrounds, they noted low or negative expectations: *'There's lots of services I know that are commissioned … but not exactly appropriate culturally or sensitive or in terms of the language, even, for people to access'* (Victor et al., 2024: 1177). People diagnosed with young-onset dementia can be decades younger than the population many memory cafés and other groups are aimed at, and understandably get frustrated when asked to reminisce about things they never experienced or listen to music from another generation. One carer told IDEAL researchers: *'There seems to be very little help, support and groups for younger people and people with early onset. Also, living in the country there's very little access to support groups or activities if you can't drive'*. This perspective adds the accessibility question: what support do you need to *get* to the support? Transport to and from services is often a barrier to access, and organisations need to think about how they expect people to attend an event or appointment.

With available options not meeting certain needs, several alternatives have developed outside mainstream services. The DEEP network of peer support groups is a good example (DEEP, 2024). However, if you live in a sparsely populated area, there may not be an in-person group accessible. While some people with dementia can get support from online meetings, this is not an option for everyone.

People affected by dementia are individuals with preferences. When we spoke to the ALWAYs group about their experiences, the importance of choice came out strongly:

KEITH: *It's about activities for those who want to join in. Often people with dementia are offered a choir, but not everyone wants to sing. They should have a range of options.*

DAVID: *Support for carers isn't personalised. I was told I could have a spa day (which I assumed was 'getting stroking' and I didn't want that!).*

While there was some giggling at David's story, it emphasises a serious point: a one-size-fits-all approach to services and support is not supportive. David was eventually offered a driving session on his local car racing circuit *'in a big BMW'*, which suited him much better.

A variety of options needs to be available to people, but as we have reiterated: how do people know what is available? One powerful banner created as part of The Unfurlings series was 'Navigating the system', the maze symbolising the confusion people can feel (Figure 10.6).

Availability covers not just whether services exist, but whether information about them is available. How do you get to know what is available? People designing services or running support groups need to promote this information and collaborate with other services in the area (see Box 10.1 for an example from Bristol, a city in the west of England). In workshops we asked: 'What do you want people in charge of dementia services to know?'. Signposting to information was a key theme, with one carer wondering, *'Who does what? Who will help me? Who will help my relative?'*; another asked for *'one person who can direct me … It is emotionally and physically exhausting chasing everyone and trying to find out what is available'* (IDEAL Programme, 2023: 10–16).

We need to broaden our horizons when thinking about services and support. How people feel about dementia, about health services, about asking for help, or about the activity on offer all affect behaviour. While dementia can be diagnosed through a set of symptoms, the experience of living with dementia is a much more varied picture. We need to help people with dementia to join the dots to find the types of services and support which would suit their individual experience.

Figure 10.6: The Kirklees DEEP group banner 'Navigating the system: Dementia support for all'.

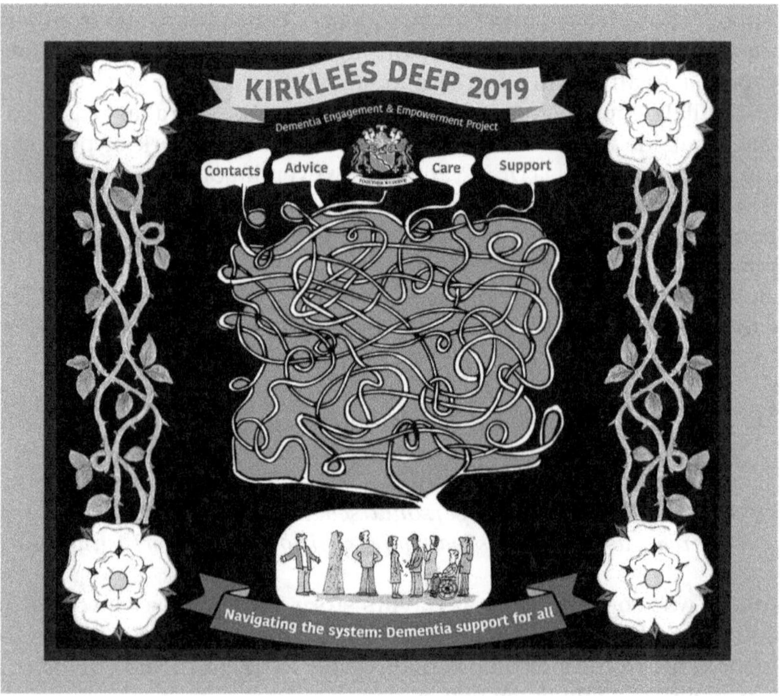

Box 10.1: An example of joined-up practice – the Bristol Dementia Wellbeing Service

The Bristol Dementia Wellbeing Service (DWS) brings together the NHS and Alzheimer's Society to deliver an innovative model of care for people living with dementia and their carers. Commissioned based on feedback from those affected by dementia, this service brings together primary and secondary care, delivering a pathway that supports people living with dementia and their carers from diagnosis, with ongoing post-diagnostic support and through to end-of-life. The service does not discharge, and people will remain with DWS throughout their dementia journey, enabling rapid access to increased support without a waiting list, and continuity of care so the individual does not need to keep retelling their story.

The service works with GPs, other health professionals, and partners across Bristol to support people with dementia with help when and where it is wanted, and in a way that suits them. Each GP practice in Bristol has a named dementia practitioner and dementia navigator. Practitioners are qualified members of the care team who work closely with the person with dementia and their GP, providing specialist memory assessments and therapeutic interventions, supporting people and their families at difficult times throughout their illness. Navigators provide practical and emotional support to people with a diagnosis and those close to them, working in a person-centred way to identify local groups and activities in the community to maintain the independence and enhance the quality of life for people with dementia. Personalised well-being plans are created, which reflect what is important to people, their plans, wishes, and support needs, now and into the future.

The service has a dedicated care home liaison team, supporting the delivery of best practice into Bristol's nursing and residential homes – whether this is working with managers, staff, or residents. Additionally, to support the vision for Bristol to be a dementia-friendly city, Community Development Co-ordinators work closely with Bristol's local communities to understand and identify barriers, overcome stigma, and support dementia awareness.

So what does this tell us about reconsidering living with dementia?

A dementia diagnosis is a starting point, and one at which people arrive with different life experiences and resources. This chapter highlights some important ideas to take forward: for those experiencing mild-to-moderate dementia, more support happens at home than in the health and social care system. Often invisible, this invaluable support needs considering and acknowledging. We have also seen the power of personalisation: a variety of services and support are needed for different diagnoses and different preferences. Finally, while funding is always an issue, we can look to models which are known to work and advice that already exists.

At our final IDEAL webinar, the ALWAYs group were asked what they thought the audience needed to take away from IDEAL. Julia said, '*Look at the person and the carer and the situation. And not just once, because what's been shown from the IDEAL project is what happens or what can happen over time*' (IDEAL Programme, 2024: 1:13:03). This might be the IDEAL model of human functioning, considering how a person's lived health evolves over time, not just through the changes dementia brings, but also those wrought by alterations in someone's social and environmental contexts.

> ### Reflections from the ALWAYs group
>
> We found the chapter clear and engaging and we were interested in the concept of 'human functioning'. Although the IDEAL data, on which the book is based, are about mild-to-moderate dementia, we think there is a lot of good advice for practitioners and providers to be aware of, understand, and proactively engage in for later in the condition. It is a certainty that the level and type of support needed, whether living alone or with a carer, will change drastically and practitioners should have a system anticipating this, based on regular communication.
>
> Additionally, the carer of the person with dementia will need a higher level of support in terms of both information and practical and emotional support. With declining energy, the inevitable progress of the dementia and, potentially, a change in the relationship between cared for and carer, increased and varied support would improve the lives of both.

> ### Key points
>
> ### Key points for people living with dementia and carers
>
> - You do not have to experience dementia alone.
> - Look at what is available to you both locally and nationally.
> - Support comes in many forms: don't be afraid to ask for what you need, to accept help when it is offered and to try different things.
>
> ### Key points for health and social care practitioners
>
> - Proactively reach out to families and share information about the services and support available.
> - Design services and support through co-production.
> - Co-operate and share information across all sources of support locally to help families navigate the landscape.

Key points for policy-makers

- Look at addressing the known barriers to accessing services.
- Mandating mapping and monitoring of dementia services would make it easier to provide people with options.
- Some patterns of support needs can be anticipated: policy could reflect the expectation to meet these needs.

 **Manifesto statement**

We want to have choices about services and support and to know about the options which are available to us.

References

Alzheimer's Society (2022) *Left to cope alone: The unmet support needs after a dementia diagnosis*. London: Alzheimer's Society. Available at: https://www.alzheimers.org.uk/about-us/policy-and-influencing/left-cope-alone-unmet-support-needs-after-dementia-diagnosis.

Bickenbach, J., Rubinelli, S., Baffone, C., et al. (2023) The human functioning revolution: implications for health systems and sciences, *Frontiers in Science*, 1(1): 1118512. Available at: https://doi.org/10.3389/fsci.2023.1118512.

DEEP (2024) *DEEP: The UK Network of Dementia Voices*. Available at: https://www.dementiavoices.org.uk/ (accessed 9 October 2024).

Goeman, D., Renehan, E. and Koch, S. (2016) What is the effectiveness of the support worker role for people with dementia and their carers? A systematic review, *BMC Health Services Research*, 16(1): 285. Available at: https://doi.org/10.1186/s12913-016-1531-2.

Henderson, C., Knapp, M., Nelis, S.M., et al. (2019) Use and costs of services and unpaid care for people with mild-to-moderate dementia: baseline results from the IDEAL cohort study, *Alzheimer's & Dementia: Translational Research and Clinical Interventions*, 5(1): 685–96.

Henley, J., Hillman, A., Jones, I.R., et al. (2023) 'We're happy as we are': the experience of living with possible undiagnosed dementia, *Ageing and Society*, 43(9): 2041–66.

IDEAL Programme (2023) *How can we improve the experience of living with dementia? A community workshop*, University of Exeter, Exeter.

IDEAL Programme (2024) *Evidence and resources from 10 years of the IDEAL programme*. YouTube. Available at: youtube.com/watch?v=buSUMTadv30&ab_channel=IDEALProgramme (accessed 9 October 2024).

National Institute for Health and Care Excellence (NICE) (2018) *Dementia: assessment, management and support for people living with dementia and their carers*, NICE Guideline NG97. Available at: https://www.nice.org.uk/guidance/ng97 (accessed 10 October 2024).

Pentecost, C., Collins, R., Stapley, S., et al. (2022) Effects of social restrictions on people with dementia and carers during the pre-vaccine phase of the COVID-19 pandemic: experiences of IDEAL cohort participants, *Health and Social Care in the Community*, 30(6): e4594–604. Available at: https://doi.org/10.1111/hsc.13863.

Quinn, C., Nelis, S.M., Martyr, A., et al. (2020) Caregiver influences on 'living well' for people with dementia: findings from the IDEAL study, *Aging and Mental Health*, 24(9): 1505–13.

Quinn, C., Hart, N., Henderson, C., et al. (2022a) Developing supportive local communities: perspectives from people with dementia and caregivers participating in the IDEAL programme, *Journal of Aging and Social Policy*, 34(6): 839–59.

Quinn, C., Pickett, J.A., Litherland, R., et al. (2022b) Living well with dementia: what is possible and how to promote it, *International Journal of Geriatric Psychiatry*, 37(1): e5627. Available at: https://doi.org/10.1002/gps.5627.

Tang, E.Y.H., Birdi, R. and Robinson, L. (2018) Attitudes to diagnosis and management in dementia care: views of future general practitioners, *International Psychogeriatrics*, 30(3): 425–30.

van Horik, J.O., Collins, R., Martyr, A., et al. (2022) Limited receipt of support services among people with mild-to-moderate dementia: findings from the IDEAL cohort, *International Journal of Geriatric Psychiatry*, 37(3): e5688. Available at: https://doi. org/10.1002/gps.5688.

Victor, C.R., van den Heuvel, E., Pentecost, C., et al. (2024) Understanding dementia in minority ethnic communities: the perspectives of key stakeholders interviewed as part of the IDEAL programme, *Dementia*, 23(7): 1172–82.

11 Meanings and methods: reflections from those involved in IDEAL

*Rachael Litherland and
Catherine Charlwood*

This chapter is different. Rather than hearing about the research evidence, we hear directly from people who worked on IDEAL. They reflect on what the experience was like, why it mattered to them, and what they will remember. Some people wrote theirs directly, others shared via a Zoom call which we wrote up with their approval. We hope that our stories give you an insight into the broader context of IDEAL.

 Linda Clare, Chief Investigator

As IDEAL closes, I ask myself: did we do what we said we would do, did we remain true to our ethos, and what legacy will we leave?

When colleagues comment on IDEAL, they usually say it is 'productive'. There is no doubt that IDEAL has been productive. Its duration has allowed us to make the most of the information people shared with us. Delivering a complex programme like IDEAL is a logistical challenge, especially when circumstances change, as with the arrival of the COVID-19 pandemic. Consequently, we did not necessarily do everything we said we would do in the way we originally proposed, and there are things we might have done better, but I believe we attempted to tackle all the questions we set ourselves.

IDEAL was built around a holistic view of dementia, going beyond medical perspectives to focus on social, relational, and emotional dimensions of living with the condition, with an ethos of collaboration and respect. We had to balance the requirement for rigour with the needs of our participants and the researchers on the ground. We also had to ask ourselves whether we were giving a sufficiently representative picture, and responsibly highlight gaps or limitations. In the early days, especially, working out our conceptual framework involved stimulating discussions, often translating the language of one discipline to another, and turning arcane terminology into accessible descriptions to find shared meaning. As time progressed, the emphasis shifted more to co-production and co-creation of resources. The idea for this book only made sense to me once we were able to frame it as a manifesto, linking IDEAL evidence with calls for action from people affected by dementia. I think this shows we stayed close to our ethos.

IDEAL has been a team effort. I feel very privileged to have worked with so many outstanding people and to have learned from their expertise, whether professional or based on experience. I want to pay tribute to everyone who has contributed to the success of IDEAL. I am especially grateful for the commitment of team members Sharon, Catherine, and Anthony, who moved with the programme when I caused considerable disruption by deciding to change university. Subsequently, there were some darker times when problems with staffing and institutional support seemed to threaten the viability of the programme, but IDEAL was too valuable to give up on, and the commitment and support of other team members got me through.

There was an added personal dimension in that dementia was very much part of my private as well as professional life throughout the programme. Spending many weekends with my mother, the third in our immediate family to develop dementia, in the nursing home where she had been admitted for end-of-life care and ended up living for 10 more years prompted much reflection on 'living well' and the scale of the challenge we face in making that a reality. Our film 'The World Turned Upside Down' still moves me to tears each time I watch it and think about how to communicate better and be a more understanding carer. With the carer role now on my horizon once again, I'm grateful for everything I've learned from IDEAL and especially from our amazing ALWAYs group members and the positive way in which they approach life with dementia or as carers.

There have been many highlights over the 10 years of IDEAL, but one of the most joyful experiences for me has been the enthusiasm of the Programme Advisory Group, which brings together professional experts and ALWAYs group members in regular meetings. They not only offered thoughtful reflections and great advice, but always valued and believed in IDEAL and its impact. I inevitably came out of those meetings feeling that what I was doing mattered.

IDEAL has forged lasting connections. Many people have engaged with our work and seem to feel it makes sense. There is enthusiasm to shape progressive approaches to improving the experience of living with dementia, and better understanding of the importance of psychological well-being and less quantifiable things like hope. The work will continue. Did we succeed in helping to change things? I hope so. Time will tell.

Nori Graham, Chair of the Programme Advisory Group, 2014–23

The experiences and problems of people living with dementia and their carers have been close to my heart throughout my professional life. It is nearly 50 years since I took part in a study looking at very similar issues conducted by

Enid Levin. At that time, we were focused on the practical problems of the carer.

Much has changed since then, but it has needed the IDEAL study to help us understand the changes. Most significantly, IDEAL has focused equally on both the person living with dementia and the carer. The study shows the importance of regular assessment of *both* the psychological and the physical health of the person living with dementia. It has demonstrated the significance of the key support services, including a single point of contact, that the carer needs. Furthermore, it has shown that carers are able to provide more effective care the better they understand the disease process. These findings are all relevant to assessment, treatment, and management. This might seem common sense to those of us who have been working in the field, but it needed to be demonstrated and provided with an evidence base. IDEAL has achieved this. What is more, these conclusions have been validated in a unique way by having people living with dementia as well as carers fully involved in the study. I think the results of the study have enormous positive implications for people living with dementia, their carers – paid and unpaid – and for all those working with them. Putting this into practice is the next challenge.

It has been my privilege to be part of IDEAL. It has been a great pleasure to work with Linda and her team. I would like to thank them and my colleagues who have served on the advisory group. We have shared a common aim: to do our best to give people living with dementia and those caring for them as good a quality of life as possible.

 ## David Scott, ALWAYs group member, 2014–23

Getting involved in research – why not? My mother-in-law had had to go into care with full-blown Alzheimer's and we had lived through the stage of her not being able to sort out her money, through to needing almost full-time care. There was an element of curiosity as well as wanting to learn more about what might result from an extended study of folks with the big 'A'. So, here comes an opportunity – join a group to contribute and learn more about how to live well with the big 'A'. A is also the first letter of the acronym ALWAYs – the name given to our involvement group – which was intent on engaging with and contributing to a large and long-lived project (IDEAL) about how to make the best of living with an incurable condition. The group was so full of existing knowledge and experience that it was an enormous privilege to share with those as carers and those actually living with the condition. Keith is our guru, having lived with dementia for over 10 years and being involved with Alzheimer's Society at the highest level. Contrast this with Jane and Julia who had lived on a day-to-day basis with close relatives in slow decline. Their insights, invaluable and insightful, provided a very practical compendium to be shared with academic researchers and others in our small group.

Early meetings were based in the former London HQ of Alzheimer's Society at Devon House with a wonderful location at Saint Katherine's Dock, a former working dock now converted to an anchorage for boats by Tower Bridge. Incidentally, Saint Catherine of Siena is the patron saint of, among others, nursing and Saint Catherine of Alexandria of students – take your pick! Much of the later business was conducted by the magical tool of Zoom, splendidly organised by our leader Rachael. The Zoom format undoubtedly helped us grow closer to each other and allowed fuller development of discussion and ideas than face-to-face good 'give-and-take'. For one thing, we could meet more frequently, which helped to keep particular elements moving along. Neither can we deny the geographical advantages since there were members across the nation from Cheshire to Northern Ireland and on to Canterbury. There was a further benefit, too: we just grew to be like a family group – good 'give-and-take' in discussion, sharing jokes and personal feelings. It was immensely productive and satisfying.

Nada Savitch, Co-Investigator and PPIE Lead, 2014–15

For the IDEAL project to be really ideal, people with dementia and carers needed to be central to everything the project did. We decided that one of the ways of involving people with dementia and carers was to set up a group. At the first meeting, researchers from the team explained the project, and we discussed the role of the group. At that stage, getting across the abstract idea of a steering group wasn't easy. But there was real enthusiasm for aiding any research that might help people with dementia live better in the future.

It was at that first meeting that the group named itself ALWAYs – with the emphasis on ASKING YOU. The way that the name was decided with everyone pitching in and agreeing made me realise that we'd got together a really great bunch of people.

The thing that I learned the most from the group is how people with very little in common can be so supportive of each other. From the very beginning, everyone was patient with others who might find it difficult to get their views across. Everyone's opinion and contributions were valued. The group didn't really need facilitation by me – everyone got together naturally and came to agreement easily.

One thing I enjoyed the most was when the group presented at a conference. Everyone – even the shyest people who had never talked in front of an audience before – were encouraged to speak: not by me, but by the group, and not by pressure, but because of the kindness shown by each and every member. It is certainly one of the kindest groups I've ever been involved with.

Allison Batchelor, ALWAYs group member, 2021–23

I joined after another piece of work called My Life, My Goals where we had co-produced a resource around goals for people with dementia. The ALWAYs group was just about to start its work on the Living with Dementia Toolkit and it was good to get involved at the beginning. I wanted to get involved because I live as well as I possibly can with dementia. I acknowledge that every day and every part of every day will be slightly different.

I think the balance of working with carers produced a much more rounded piece of work that would benefit the person living with a dementia diagnosis but also the carers. I did enjoy working with them very much.

For example, we had a long discussion about risk. If that bit of the Toolkit had only been produced by people with dementia or only produced by carers it would have been a completely different outcome. You were able to listen to what the carers were saying, and they, very willingly, listened to what we were saying as well. I think there was a good compromise that both parties were really happy with. There was no awkwardness at all, and yet there were a lot of differences in that topic. But we respect each other's opinions. The facilitators have made it very smooth. It's always enjoyable, it's never a chore to do.

I don't know if we have just been extremely lucky but there have never been any issues. It's not always the case with other groups!

I love looking on my whiteboard in the morning and seeing there is an ALWAYs meeting. It gives me a real sense of purpose. It gives me the feeling that I still have something to contribute, that I am making a difference. Following the dementia diagnosis, I thought my opinion was never going to be asked for again. I am so unbelievably proud to see some of the work I have been part of.

I won't settle for any other ways of being involved from now on! I know what works. I know that it can work.

Paula Brown, Research Delivery Psychologist, Nottinghamshire Healthcare NHS Trust, 2014–20

I have met with and come to know many families living with dementia who have given their valuable time and support to two particular studies – the IDEAL study and Effective Home Support in Dementia Care. Both studies involved asking people who were currently living with dementia about their views, experiences, and ideas for future support. Specifically, the studies asked questions to gain information and insight into what aspects of everyday life were working well, what could be improved, and what people's preferences were for future support and services.

Visiting people to talk about dementia research, when many of them had only received their diagnosis in recent months, was initially daunting. I had previously worked clinically with people living with dementia, but not asked them about research so soon after being diagnosed.

On a personal level, I experienced a rollercoaster of emotions, as during this time I was caring for my grandma who had recently been diagnosed with dementia, as well as witnessing the changes in a friend's life as they were coping with a diagnosis of young-onset dementia. Friends and family members had reported that in the weeks following their diagnosis, they were still coming to terms with the news, and were finding it hard to distinguish what was working well or what their needs were or might be in the future.

However, despite my early wobbles, I was amazed at just how many people told me that getting involved in research helped them. They felt it enabled them to learn more about dementia, that they benefited from sharing their initial observations on the immediate effects of dementia on their lives, and that they were more empowered and in control of what the future might hold for them and their loved ones.

For five years I visited participants for lengthy sessions, with interviews and assessments involving some direct and personal questions. This led to some special bonds, as I came to know more about their everyday lives, relationships, and well-being.

I am truly grateful for this experience, and feel it was a tremendous privilege. Every day, while working on these studies, I was fascinated by the individual life stories that were shared with me; clearly, dementia is only a small part of what is often an incredible personal story. Over the years, hearing about and observing, what for many was a significant deterioration in daily functioning, was immensely upsetting. Yet, alongside this I also witnessed things that were uplifting – the skills and abilities demonstrated, and the innovative adaptations made to life by families was simply inspirational.

The strength and generosity of these participants to share their experiences, especially in challenging times, is why these studies were able to create and develop materials and resources to help others who will live with dementia in the future – or as IDEAL states, to 'live well' despite the challenges.

An essential part of research is sharing not only the results, but any resources developed by study teams, with participants and staff. For me, this makes research open and accessible to all. The Living with Dementia Toolkit from IDEAL is based on five themes which research shows have an impact on people's ability to live well and feel good. What it means to feel good is different for everyone, so the toolkit is a way of supporting people with dementia and their carers to find out more about the areas of importance to them. Each area has several parts with short videos, top tips and strategies, links to further resources, and (my favourite) good examples of 'how to' using real-life positive stories.

This reflection was originally published as a blog entitled 'Research Delivery: working on dementia studies – my personal experience and sharing the outcomes' on the Institute of Mental Health, Nottingham, blog.

Toby Williamson, Independent Health and Social Care Consultant and member of the Programme Advisory Group, 2014–23

The IDEAL research project has gone on for so long that I have difficulty recalling when I was invited to be a member of its advisory group. I think it was pretty much from the start. At that time, I was Head of Later Life at the Mental Health Foundation, a UK social research, development, and policy charity. I had led several small-scale research projects involving people with dementia and family carers about quality-of-life issues, as well as trying to help promote the voice of people with dementia through initiatives such as the Dementia Engagement and Empowerment Project (DEEP) network. I was also involved in various ways trying to influence national dementia policy. I guess that combination was seen to be useful for IDEAL's advisory group and I hope it proved to be the case.

In my experience it is amazing, and brilliant, for a large-scale dementia research project to have gone on as long as IDEAL. I cannot speak more highly of any major research project that I'm aware of than IDEAL. Dementia has no cure and treatments are still limited in efficacy and the types of dementia they can be used for. It is therefore essential that we understand what supports the well-being of people affected by dementia (including family carers) on a scale big enough, and for long enough, to provide solid evidence that can be used to shape policy, services, and practice. It is also very important that we have a better balance between social and biomedical research, which is still too heavily tilted towards the latter. IDEAL does all of that, with a prolific output, as well as ticking the boxes about being methodologically 'robust' research. But IDEAL does other things as well.

It's good to see the growing acceptance of meaningful and properly supported involvement of people with lived experience in dementia research projects. But doing this involvement correctly requires expertise and experience in its own right. The team at IDEAL understand this and recognise this is best done in partnership; through Innovations in Dementia and the ALWAYs group of people with dementia and family carers, the involvement seems to have been exemplary, though it is sad that not all members of the group lived long enough to see IDEAL get to where it is today.

Yet IDEAL has gone even further, supporting a whole range of brilliant and creative spin-offs that include practical resources for people living with dementia, and to my mind, the best visual celebration of living with dementia, in the form of the Banners for Hope and Change. IDEAL's provision of information during the COVID-19 pandemic was another great example of putting research into practice, and I was pleased to be able to help make this information more accessible for people affected by dementia from Black, Asian, and minority ethnic communities. Although IDEAL is not explicitly focused on rights, equality, diversity, and inclusion, its evidence provides great support for all of them.

Since 2016, I have worked as a freelance consultant and I am so glad that I am still involved with IDEAL as part of the advisory group. Through teaching, training, and writing, I point people towards IDEAL and I would encourage others to do the same. I've now become a carer for my mum who has dementia, so IDEAL's output is now of great personal use. Well done and thank you to Linda, the researchers and the wider team, and all the IDEAL research participants, for such a major contribution to how we understand and can positively support quality of life for people affected by dementia.

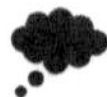 Jacqui Bingham, ALWAYs group member, 2021–23

I got involved in the ALWAYs group because it's a group where we make things happen. The group always gels from the very beginning. Everybody always understands each other and where they are coming from, whether they be carers or not. We all just seem to slot in and it's so easy to work together.

Many people do not understand dementia, they just don't get it, or want to get it. So for me to be in a group with people who get it is so wonderful. It also makes me feel that it is not just me. I'm accepted in the group even though I feel certain things. And the carers in the group also understand, very well, how I feel.

Before the meetings, I am so excited. It's something to look forward to and be connected to. I'm not connected to anybody else. Connection is a huge thing for me. I get it here in this group and with IDEAL. I've always been able to say what I feel. I've been called difficult over the years. But when I express my opinions in this group, people respect them, and that is a huge thing for me.

I feel very proud to see the work we have done together. I also feel very connected and included. If I feel like that when we were working on it, it has to extend further to the people who are using our resources such as the Living with Dementia Toolkit.

I feel brilliant after our meetings – a bit tired but a satisfied tiredness. The way this group works, it has brought me to a stage where I am choosy about what I get involved in. I wanted to be involved in everything at one stage. But I don't need that. I want to be in groups that make me feel happy.

Catherine Quinn, Co-Investigator, 2014–23

For me, being part of IDEAL has been an extraordinary opportunity. I did not realise at the start just how big the study would become, particularly in terms of the range of outputs (who knew we would end up with all these banners or a song). We've had a unique opportunity to work with a large group of co-investigators, collaborators, and the ALWAYs group over a long period of time. This has meant we have had the opportunity to develop as a team. The study has introduced me to the complexities of cohort data collection but also the importance of ensuring each individual's different experiences are heard. Many of the topics we have looked at in the study were, at the time, under-explored in people with dementia. I hope that one thing we have shown with this study is that you can ask people with dementia for their perspective on issues such as their quality of life.

I have very much learned from working with the ALWAYs group; they have been a reassuring guiding presence throughout the study. I was there in the meeting when we came up with their name and that identity has been hugely important to the study. They are fantastic ambassadors for IDEAL and we've had some fun times together, such as the day we spent in London recording the ALWAYs group video. One of the things they have constantly reminded us about is the importance of the study in raising awareness of issues affecting the quality of life of people with dementia and their carers. It was lovely to have their involvement in my chapters in this book, guiding me on what topics to focus on.

In current times, where it feels like the focus is predominantly on the development of even earlier diagnosis through things like biomarkers or the search for a cure, it can be easy to forget the importance of improving support for people living with dementia now. Improving 'care' is equally as important as finding a 'cure'. I hope that one of the lasting legacies of this study and this book is that we've been able to raise awareness of the many different things that can affect people's quality of life and how important access to good support is for both people with dementia and carers. We can't expect people to live well without the right support being in place.

 Julia Burton, ALWAYs group member, 2014–23

My first encounter with dementia was with my mother, Stella, who died with dementia nearly 20 years ago. I wanted to learn and do more about dementia and became involved with Alzheimer's Society, volunteering in a local memory café and as a lay member of the Alzheimer's Society Research Network.

We met regularly at Alzheimer's Society buildings in London, during the early years of IDEAL and then near King's Cross but latterly, largely on Zoom. Some of us were able to meet up in Exeter after the Living with Dementia Toolkit launch in November 2021 and afterwards for a meal together: it was exciting and delightful to share hugs in the real world. It has been a privilege to be part of this dynamic group of people with dementia and people who are or have been caregivers. All of us have the shared purpose of improving life for those experiencing dementia, a mission to find out by asking them what matters, a commitment to doing our best to spread research findings and get outputs implemented. ALWAYs – Action on Living Well, Asking You! We've become a productive and happy group, tackling big issues with honesty and humour, feeling valued and validated. Just writing this brings a wide smile to my face.

My own involvement has developed from reviewing documents and questionnaires for their accessibility to being involved in 'live' IDEAL events. My highlights include co-presenting the end-of-study symposium for the original IDEAL project in 2018 at Friends House, Euston; the making of the 'Meet the ALWAYs group' film in London in 2018 that is still being shown as an example of public participation in research (Joff Winterhart, graphic artist, was one of the production team and we all treasure the individual caricatures he did for us on the day); casting alongside the director, Paul Jepson, for the theatre production 'The World Turned Upside Down' held in January 2022 in Exeter, and going on to shape the documentary film.

Most importantly, it is the focused, critical, and creative teamwork, fostered by IDEAL and supported by Innovations in Dementia, resulting in the co-production of the Living with Dementia Toolkit and this book that is the best bit for me. The shape and content of both of these permanent products have been influenced and sometimes inspired by our suggestions. Along with other IDEAL outputs, these form pioneering examples of the success achieved by shared pairing of lived experience and academia remaining actively involved together during a long research process.

I'm proud and delighted that our lived experience is acknowledged by IDEAL as a valuable part of communicating findings. Through the years, apart from the sheer pleasure of working alongside such a dedicated, open-minded team of ALWAYs colleagues and IDEAL researchers, I've learned so much: built up my knowledge and understanding of dementia and of research generally; been inspired by the people I've met to maintain my positive attitude to facing up to life's challenges; and encouraged by IDEAL to believe that the quality of life for people affected by dementia can and will be improved.

 ## Emma Walter, Administrator, 2020–23

My desire to work in the field of dementia was sparked by a family history of dementia, in particular the impact it has had on the family since my mum's diagnosis. I had previously worked as an events manager, which I enjoyed, but the desire for a deeper sense of job satisfaction increased as time went on. IDEAL has afforded me the opportunity to plug that gap!

Through the plethora of IDEAL outputs – particularly the creative ones – I have experienced a different view of living with dementia, a more positive one, a more hopeful one. Some of the people with lived experience that have been part of IDEAL have been truly inspiring. Their unshakable desire to change perceptions and experiences is astounding; their desire to wring every drop of positivity from their experiences is wonderful.

There have been times when IDEAL has made me consider my own attitude, behaviour, and naivety about dementia, often thinking that I wish I could have seen this or read that or behaved differently, when my family were experiencing particularly difficult times.

I hope that the legacy of IDEAL continues long into the future and that many, many families feel supported and heartened by IDEAL and all those that have been part of it.

 ## Keith Oliver, ALWAYs group member, 2014–23

I've been in the project since the beginning. I see the IDEAL project itself, and the ALWAYs group, as very much entwined together, but with an element of separation as well. IDEAL has been far more than the ALWAYs group but the ALWAYs group has been a significant part of it.

IDEAL gave me insight into how the researcher was going to formulate the questions to ask other people with dementia. I'd never had that privilege of working with researchers in this way. It was a learning experience which I enjoyed. To see the project grow and emerge in the way it did was immensely satisfying, rewarding, and interesting. All of the opportunities I've been given, to speak alongside eminent academics and professionals has been great for my self-confidence and self-esteem. I've never felt on the periphery of it – I've always felt part of a team. It's partly them, and partly me, and partly the subject matter. They wanted to engage in the way they have, they had a commitment to enabling me, and people like me, to share the space with them. There's been a definite sense of sharing, and a definite sense of equality within the project, which is quite rare. Mutual respect has always been at the centre of our collaboration.

And there has been a lot of opportunity, the masterclass, the film, the opera and the play, the launch of the Living with Dementia Toolkit, speaking at conferences about IDEAL – Swansea to Chicago! It has been an enormous part of my life for nine years. I feel part of IDEAL.

It has been kept alive in my mind because of the frequency of our meetings. I've backed off from some projects because they haven't been able to do that and I don't get that sense of co-created ownership, like I do in IDEAL.

IDEAL is quite unique in what it set out to achieve. IDEAL gives you the evidence to help people to live well with dementia and to show, with support and opportunity, to go some way to achieving that. When I got involved, I didn't know where it was going to lead. The academics and those involved didn't either! We were learning together. This was an important ingredient in a successful research project, we could work it out together.

In IDEAL and ALWAYs, there has been continuity but also renewal and replacement. We have grown and learned together.

This book is part of our legacy. We want this project to have made a difference to the lives of people with dementia and family carers. It's not just what we found out, but how it will be used.

🌳 Monica Cheeseman, ALWAYs group member, 2014–23

Hello, I am Monica, and I live in a village on the Hampshire-Surrey border. I have been volunteering at Alzheimer's Society for the past 10 years. This means that along with many other such volunteers, I read lay proposals from potential researchers hoping to research the cause, cure, or care for people with dementia.

I joined the ALWAYs group as an ex-carer. Over the years there has been a good bond between the two researchers we now meet with, on Zoom on a regular basis even throughout COVID-19! There are four people with dementia and four carers. We listen and all learn from each other, especially that no two people are the same and we have a laugh at times. We have met with DEEP groups in Manchester, spoken on Zoom with students in Exeter and answered questions from our experience and other great connections.

I was a carer for my aunt who had Alzheimer's. I repatriated her from Cyprus. I run a coffee morning in our village once a month (up to 40 people attend) and a monthly Singing for Fun Group. In both groups we have folk with dementia, all very different, male and female. I have supported Jane, whose daughter lives in Canada; John and his wife, Brenda; and Cliff who had frontotemporal dementia with very poor communication, but who loved to walk. I walked with him when I could as his wife was unwell. I still meet with people with dementia regularly. I also learn much from the monthly Zoom meetings with our wonderful, enthusiastic researchers, Rachael and Cathy – what a joy! So much discussion takes place between us all to collaborate the Living with Dementia Toolkit and now this book.

I always remember sitting with my aunt, her communication was limited or generally non-existent. She gave me a lovely sense of appreciation. She knew who had brought her back to her English home and provided her comfort and care. For her and those I know, I continue to share knowledge and gain from them all – what a privilege.

 Chris Norris, ALWAYs group member, 2021–23

IDEAL's involvement with people with dementia has been phenomenal – so many organisations don't come close. It is co-production all the time and you feel very valued. It is IDEAL!

They give us involvement at every stage. Firstly, I participated as part of the study. That was very friendly. They made sure of the little things to ensure it was easy to participate, things like they checked beforehand that I was still happy to do it, and they checked with my wife that she was happy to do it. This was every time that the interviews were carried out. This enabled us to be comfortable and relaxed on every visit. So, we didn't just plough into it. It felt genuine. It felt like a worthwhile project to help create a much greater understanding around the experience of living with dementia to help people cope with their future and to help me as well. They have dug deep. Subsequently, I haven't come across any research that comes near it.

Then I got involved in the ALWAYs group and the Living with Dementia Toolkit. I wanted to take it further. I wanted to help people to do things for themselves and to achieve a better life.

It is really important that we create resources that are alive, easily accessible, relatable, enjoyable, educational, and that leap off the page for the person using them. This was achieved in spades! Not boring or a challenge to plough through but so good that the person using it wants to come back time and time again. Our work is always a laugh, it's an opportunity to have a good chuckle, which allows us to be slightly off the wall in what we say. It's very fulfilling from that point of view. The whole thing is just so proactive to get the best out of the people taking part.

In this IDEAL book, it is not just academics giving their opinion but it's the living 'lab rats' that are doing so as well! We pull things apart, strip the meat off it, and put more meat back on!

I have enjoyed hearing other people's opinions. You get variety. We have fun. I feel my views are listened to and taken on board.

IDEAL gives you hope eternal that changes are taking place and that they will take place. On the back of what we have learned, we are going to make sure that change takes place.

Catherine Henderson, Research Fellow, 2014–23

I joined as an economic evaluator, and from the beginning I enjoyed working with all the members of the team, many of whom are still involved today. We had many planning meetings in the early days, so there were plenty of opportunities to get to know people. I particularly appreciated having the chance to meet researchers from a wide range of different disciplines. I have worked closely with the team along the way, for instance in training fieldworkers, working on papers and the 'data linkage' project. This last was an effort to link some health records data from UK health statistics agencies to data from participants who had given consent for this. It has been a bit of a saga but suffice to say that our 'data linkage' project took nine years to progress and would never have got that far without the determined efforts of Linda, IDEAL programme manager Sharon, and current programme manager Claire.

I have really appreciated IDEAL's public involvement and engagement efforts over the years, in particular the opportunity to meet members of the ALWAYs group and to make connections with people living with dementia and carers of people living with dementia during the programme's public webinar series. IDEAL has also offered a great opportunity to work with policy-makers from Alzheimer's Society. The research I've been involved in has been enriched by the support and advice of these experts.

Like so many people, I had a parent who developed Alzheimer's disease. My mother was diagnosed around the time IDEAL was beginning, so I had my own experience of watching a loved one live their life with dementia. I go back to that experience a lot in my research.

I've learned so much from everyone I've worked with on IDEAL and learned a lot by working on the IDEAL data. But there's still more to learn.

Jane Ward, ALWAYs group member, 2014–23

My experience with dementia began with my late mum, Ella, receiving her diagnosis in 2007. Mum had always had a positive outlook, and I was incredibly lucky that she mostly retained this. Inevitably, she started losing large parts of herself and we did have some really tough times, but she wanted to continue enjoying her life and to stay independent as long as possible and I have some incredible memories. I sometimes struggled to cope with my caring role – balancing mum's needs and my own. A breakthrough for me came when I found out about the Alzheimer's Society Research Network. Getting involved enabled me to feel I was taking back some control; I learned a lot about dementia and I also had the hope that we could be part of making a difference for the future.

I joined the ALWAYs group just after I lost mum. I had also just started working on the Dementia Friendly Communities Project, so research aimed at understanding how people can live well with dementia was of great interest. I had no idea back then just how incredible the experience would be. Of course, it's been great working with the wonderful researchers on the project and contributing to its outputs, but this project has been about so much more.

Initially, our activities with the ALWAYs group were fairly typical PPIE (Patient and Public Involvement), but we quickly started to form a special bond within the group. The membership of the group has changed a little over the years, but it has always retained a special and unique feeling of belonging and trust. The respect we have for each other and confidence to speak honestly meant we really came to understand each other's viewpoints, especially in the differences between the experience of having dementia and that of caring for someone who does.

We've also had the trust to open ourselves to wonderful new experiences. These opportunities were completely unexpected, and I've loved them and the laughter they have brought, but most of all I've valued working on them with my great friends, the ALWAYs group.

Catherine Charlwood, Research Translation and Impact Manager, 2021–23

I come from an unusual background, with three degrees in literature. Alongside my PhD on memory in poetry, my grandma was living with Alzheimer's disease and I was discovering dementia, and its ripple effect across a family. When this role was advertised, it was a serendipitous alignment of personal and professional interests.

I've been at the interface between IDEAL and the wider world of the many people and organisations who could put our findings to use. This has people with dementia and carers themselves at its heart, but also community groups, healthcare professionals, students of all ages, teachers and researchers, NHS managers, and all the way up the chain to policy-makers. I'm incredibly fortunate to have this role (few such positions are ever funded), because I can dedicate my time to sharing insights and resources that stand to help others. Academic research is an exacting career, full of disappointments and reminders to try harder and do better. One of the things I love about my job is that I get to remind researchers of the 'wins': how their work has changed things for somebody else. My monthly impact round-up emails end 'Stay safe and well, and know that what you do matters' – it does matter, but we too easily forget that.

Much of my work has been with the ALWAYs group and many more people with lived experience. It's a privilege to be entrusted with people's stories and to learn from their wealth of knowledge. I've become an evangelist for co-production, because it improves research so much, offers a remarkable return on investment, and it's fun. The human warmth and connection gained really puts the work into perspective. To researchers, I say, co-production meetings are incredibly satisfying because there's a drive towards decision-making: co-production offers a world of productivity!

Creating the Living with Dementia Toolkit was particularly special. Beginning from the foundation of research evidence, the co-production of the whole resource was characterised by an extreme amount of giggles and goodwill. While the process transpired to be quite tricky (trying to have everyone record their own voices in our various homes across the UK), I'm proud that the voiceover to the toolkit animation is, in fact, our voices rather than that of a professional. The importance of personalisation has come out so strongly from IDEAL, so it's fitting that our largest public resource comes with a lot of personality behind it.

Rachael Litherland, Co-Investigator and PPIE Lead, 2016–23

I have had the treasured role of supporting the ALWAYs group since 2016. Or maybe they have supported me?

For many years, we met face-to-face in a familiar space in London, arriving from various locations to our regular meeting room in King's Cross alongside the Grand Union Canal. Our temporary, blue-tacked ALWAYs group signs were emblazoned around the venue, directing us always to the heart of IDEAL, keeping us on track (and locating the toilets!). People with dementia, carers and me … a bit of a lion's den of lived knowledge and expertise that IDEAL researchers walked into!

We commented, tweaked, amended, created, and turned some things upside down! Action on Living Well: Asking You. The ALWAYs group have lived and worked by this honorific. Research training, interview questions, creative banners, films, presentations, data analysis, and a new measure of living with dementia – everything is different because of input by the ALWAYs group.

It worked because we built relationships, trust, and ideas with each other, but also with the researchers. We became part of the IDEAL team, and wonderfully, the team welcomed us with open arms. Patient and Public Involvement, an arm of good research projects, became co-production and co-design.

COVID-19 moved us on to online meetings. What we lost from our physical contact we recreated within the safety of Zoom rooms. It also gave us the opportunity to meet more regularly and to work more continuously on co-produced projects such as the Living with Dementia Toolkit.

Ten years has been a long time for a group to exist. We've had loads of fun. We've worked very hard. We have had deep, deep discussions, people have supported each other, respectfully challenged, cried together, and laughed together. So much laughter!

We have also experienced sadnesses and losses as things have changed for ALWAYs members and members have died. We hold those names and experiences close to the group: they remain important members of the ALWAYs group, even when we no longer can see them.

I inherited my role with the group from my colleague Nada (whose reflection you can read previously). For this experience I will forever be grateful – ALWAYs.

12 Call to action: a dementia manifesto

*Rachael Litherland, Catherine Charlwood
and members of the ALWAYs group*

Each of the chapters of this book, apart from the first and the previous one, ends in a manifesto point. This chapter draws these together in the same order in which they appeared in the earlier chapters, and not in order of importance. Although the focus of this chapter is people directly affected by dementia, there are many lessons for life here which are useful for all of us.

If the lives of people with dementia and those supporting them are going to improve, we need to see changes. We restate each manifesto statement with indicators of how it could be achieved. These are not prioritised for importance: all of them matter. While the voices of all ALWAYs group members are represented here – people living with dementia and carers alike – we have chosen to use 'we', the first-person collective pronoun, as the voice of people living with dementia, because we believe this voice too often goes unheard.

> **1. We are all different: we want you to find out about us so you can best enable us to live with dementia.**

- Give us time to explain what is happening. Health and social care professionals should not rush us. This might mean offering a 'double appointment' so that we have enough time to express ourselves. We may need different methods of contact: some of us can no longer use the phone. Record our preferences for contacting us and support us to keep in touch with you.
- Acknowledge that we are all different and do not fit into one box: treat us as individuals. We are as diverse as the rest of the population. Some of us have carers, others live alone, others have carers at a distance (across counties, countries, or continents), and not all of us have children. We may identify as LGBTQ+; we may or may not have a partner. We do not necessarily share the same cultural background or want to listen to the same music. Respect our individuality.
- To the professionals who work with us, find out about our backgrounds and our lives and check in from time to time.

- It is hurtful to be told 'you don't look like you have dementia' or 'you don't sound like you have dementia', even when people might think that is a compliment. You are denying our existence and telling us that we do not conform to your expectations of us. At worst, it sounds like we are being called a fraud and could burden us with guilt.

- Learn about the different types of dementia. Lots of people mix up Alzheimer's disease and dementia: 'Alzheimer's disease' is **not** synonymous with 'dementia'; it is one type of dementia. Dementia is also not all about memory. Some of us have quite different challenges. Recognise that we might have different types of dementia and respond to us accordingly. Do not expect us to conform to your expectation.

- As Wayne, our friend living alone with young-onset dementia, said: '*Just because someone's got dementia doesn't mean – **it really doesn't mean** – that it's memory that's messing up their day. Your senses can be an absolute nightmare*'.

> **2. We want to live in a way that suits us and be supported to adapt to changes.**

- There are 'dos' and 'don'ts' for this one. Do offer us tolerance, support, and understanding; do listen to us; do try and take on board what we are saying to you (this is more than listening – it is acting on the listening). Do understand that some days we live as well as we can and other days it is much, **much** harder. This day-to-day variability is common to dementia of all types and at different stages. Do not write us off; do not patronise us. Do not try and fit us into one box – do not even try to fit us into the same box which suited us yesterday, or this morning. We have debunked the 'one box' approach in the previous manifesto point: we might not have a carer, and our dementia might be less about memory issues than other things. Dementia is progressive, but while we expect there to be changes, we still want to be supported to live in a way that suits us. There needs to be a presumption of life rather than a rush to assuming we are in a risky decline. Do not be too quick to reduce our independence – think about how we can be enabled to maintain some independence.

- Forewarned is forearmed: some of the changes dementia brings can be anticipated – tell us about them. What is likely to happen? What can we do about it? What can you do to help? Keep checking in about the changes. Dementia is not a condition where a one-off approach will work.

- As an example of the above, professionals and support organisations should introduce the topic of incontinence early. Do not allow this to be a taboo subject and do not wait until we are in crisis to have that conversation.

- Think broadly about changes where we might need help adapting. The changes dementia brings are the most obvious, but a change in our carer's health (if we have one) has a big impact; a change in our environment, such as an activity stopping through lack of funding or having to move house because – through young-onset dementia and stopping working – we cannot manage the mortgage, can rock our world. Help us to understand what is happening and how we can cope.

> **3. The well-being of the carer is as important as that of the person living with dementia: we want both to be supported.**

- Not everyone has an unpaid or family carer, but most people have someone who supports them. Carers and supporters are important.
- It is as simple as this: if you support the carer, they can support us; if you do not support the carer, both of us fall.
- In becoming a carer, people must often take on new roles or tasks which they are not used to. This could be becoming (solely) responsible for the household finances, keeping the garden tidy, or taking on the cooking. These extra 'asks' can be overwhelming and many of them could be anticipated. We encourage anyone who supports carers to have a checklist of tasks which might fall to carers and talk to them about how they are managing. For instance, if a carer is taking over responsibility for the gardening but either has no interest in gardening or would physically struggle to garden, directing them to local gardening services could be an important lifeline. Ask yourself, 'What has this person got to do now they are a carer? And how are we going to help that person do those things to keep life as calm and enjoyable as possible for both?'
- Remember that 'new' tasks can also differ by gender. Jane met a male carer who said, '*I was 73 when I bought my first bra*' (for his wife). He struggled as it was all new to him. Another male carer washed his wife's hair following a perm because he did not know this was unnecessary.
- Talk to the carer and the person with dementia as individuals and then as a partnership. Understanding the viewpoint of each – and the potential differences – will enable you to help them relate to each other.
- At times it is appropriate that support is offered solely to the carer to meet their needs, but at other times it is equally important to offer support to both the carer and the person they are caring for.
- Do not take the word of the carer as the definitive view. While the carer can tell you how they see or feel about a situation, they cannot tell you how we see or feel about it. For instance, carers are more likely than we are to think about risk and keeping us safe. Carers feel a heightened sense of responsibility and it is easy for them to overcompensate.
- Document that someone is a carer in their GP records and use that knowledge to check in on how they are coping. Do not allow a carer to get to crisis point: it is always possible to step in before someone reaches crisis point.

> **4. We want to be included as active members of our communities and wider society, with opportunities to grow and maintain meaningful social connections.**

- Speak to us without a pre-conceived script: have a conversation with us – who knows what we will discover together if we are both allowed to speak.
- There is a difference between hearing and listening. Actively listen to what we say, enable us to express our preferences, and respond to them. Think about what we might not be saying.
- The most important thing is to be listened to. Do not presume that someone with dementia cannot communicate for themselves. This is as true in a café as in a doctor's surgery.
- We need support from banks, shops, and transport services to carry on with our everyday life. The support available should not be just dementia-related, but part of an inclusive society: enable us to go to the pub, a gig, the theatre. Help us use public transport (where available).
- We want to relate to our communities and societies as people, not just with our 'dementia' hat on. Dementia-friendly activities are good and important, but also think about how we can be included in 'normal' situations, like a church service.
- Invite us to events, include us within activities, and introduce us to other people: we want to be involved in our communities.
- Part of living in a community is living in a safe environment – not just physically safe, but scam safe too. Make sure we know how to avoid scams: give us reminders we can stick on or by our phones and computers, or on our front doors. Remember that frauds can be very sophisticated and might target a skillset we acquired more recently, such as using a mobile phone or the internet, and these newer skills can be on shaky ground with our dementia. Help us to find out about services and devices which can protect us.

> **5. Relationships matter: we want to be supported to build and maintain our relationships.**

- Take the medical framing out of relationships. The people in front of you do not just relate to each other as person with dementia and carer. First and foremost, we might be lifelong partners, father and son, or best friends. Try to ask yourself: how could you, or would you, help if dementia was not part of the picture? This kind of social relationship support might be just what is needed, rather than another reminder that a lot of the time we are categorised in medical terms. Remember that these two people are living a life together, rather than a condition.

- Not everyone is in a conventional partnership. Do not make assumptions about relationships. Every carer needs help, and every relationship needs support to maintain the human connections behind it rather than merely dealing with the medical condition.
- Companionship is important: having somebody experience dementia alongside you can be comforting. We may also gain a bit of confidence from being supported by someone who knows us. Recognise the power of this and the importance of keeping us connected to each other.
- Remember that not everything has to be done together. We talked about how carers can feel under pressure to keep us active and always doing something. However, sometimes we need to rest and it is alright to let us sleep; that is not a cause for worry or for guilt. Help carers find ways to have their own 'me time'.

> **6. We want to be encouraged and enabled to do as much as we can.**

- Take an individual approach: some people might find it easier to have someone with them on outings; others might not. Ask us: what do **you** need to be able to do this activity?
- Stress or anxiety can affect our ability to complete everyday tasks. Help us to stay calm as we attempt things or encourage us to try again when the situation is less time-pressured, for instance.
- Do not just **tell** us what we can do, **show** us by putting us in touch with peer support. Someone already living with dementia is very knowledgeable and can offer us a variety of ideas on how to live life.
- Give us support to do the things we used to do by making things easier. For instance, you could take the components for a recipe out of the fridge and cupboards, so that we are not hunting for them.
- Be a helper, not a doer: do not replace us and our participation in daily activities. Manageable challenge and patience are our bywords.
- What practical help can you offer? Sometimes, the issue is nothing to do with memory. For instance, one man struggled to make a cup of tea, but when he was asked why he could not do it, it was because the kettle was too heavy. Once he got a lighter kettle, he could make hot drinks again.
- To the people around us: please be someone who allows us to choose which activities we want to participate in and support us in that choice; do not choose for us. We shared stories of peers whose carers decided for them whether they would go on a trip, or be in a choir session, and we agreed that it upset us. Do not close us off from the outside world.

- We want to ban the word 'should'. We are often told we 'should' do certain things (and not others). What you think we 'should' do, though, might be something we would hate. 'Should' places the responsibility back on the shoulders of the person who you are trying to help without giving them the support to go with it. A better word is 'could'.

> **7. We want all our health needs to be treated in a way that fits with our requirements, regardless of age.**

- Offer us appointments and encourage us to make use of health services. We do not like 'making a fuss'; we might not remember what we need and if we have to ask several times for what we need we are likely to give up. You can encourage us to say what we want to say.
- We may live with multiple health conditions which interact. Help us to look after our health holistically rather than trying to treat each part of our health as if the other parts do not exist. For instance, prescribing a pill for high blood pressure relates to dementia, because we need to remember how to get it and then to take it.
- Seeing the same GP at appointments helps us enormously. We can build up trust and they will know the narrative of the whole picture of our health, rather than starting from scratch each time.
- Really listen to what we are telling you. Do not pre-judge who is coming through the door and the treatments we need based on our medical notes. Please let us speak for ourselves and not initially through a caregiver.
- We think few people realise that dementia is often accompanied by other health conditions. Raising public awareness of this could help people be more understanding of the challenges we and our carers face.
- We talked about how generic some 'helpful' suggestions can be, especially for maintaining or improving mental health. These suggestions easily fall into the 'should' trap we mentioned. Jacqui gave the example of being told she should go out into nature, but she does not want to. However, when she is on her mobility scooter and on a mission, she appreciates hearing the birds and seeing the trees from a position of comfort.
- 'Regardless of age' is an important phrase to keep in mind because people can have bad age-related experiences at various ages. For people with younger-onset dementia, do not disregard us because we are young. For older people, do not write off our health concerns as age-related: there is no age limit on wanting to feel well, or pain-free.
- It is very difficult when someone does not want to acknowledge their health problems and we recognise this happens. If professionals can treat health holistically, though, and ask about a range of things and build up a rapport once we have made it through the door, we think that could help people get support sooner.

> **8. We want our well-being to be supported and to be seen for who we really are.**

- This is one area where it is vital to be conscious of what the person in front of you needs and wants: mood is highly individual. If you force on us what you think we 'should' do, we will end up feeling worse. Enhance the good days and support the bad.

- Look beyond the immediate presentation: our charm and good manners are socially learned. We seem like we are fine, but we might not be.

- *'Ask us about how we feel: our worries and our fears. And check in from time to time'.* These wise words from Julia could apply equally to the network around us in our local community, as well as to any health and social care professionals working with us.

- Health and social care practitioners need to share information and to be consistent in their ability and willingness to support us. If this means changing policy so that systems can talk to each other, then we are asking policy-makers to change the rules: anything which brings health and social care closer together will benefit us. We should not be allowed to fall through the gap because, for instance, the geographical boundaries of the health and social services differ.

- Look past the condition we are now diagnosed with or that we are talking about and find out about our background, history, where we have been, things we have done – sometimes, when you look into it, it is personality and not dementia which causes a challenge. We might always have been a bit outspoken or controversial; we might always have preferred our own company as a child, and still do now. You have to dig a little deeper. If you know us well, you can more readily identify a change which could be due to an infection, or to medication.

- In previous statements, we have looked at connecting with other people. It is easier to connect people to other people than to connect someone to themselves. How can you help us connect to things we as individuals are interested in? How can you help us take on personal challenges? How can you lead us to ways in which we might support ourselves to achieve well-being?

- Family and friends are likely to notice changes and are more able to identify what we really want because they know us, and they have grown alongside us on this journey. It is a high-level skill to be able to identify what we need and who we really are if you are a professional carer coming in and out. We would like professional carers to have some dementia-specific training and we can help by having some details about us and our lives available.

> **9. We want to have choices about services and support and to know about the options which are available to us.**

- Provide information about things you know about. Remember that we might be reeling from the news of a diagnosis and need some help navigating the way forward: let us know who and what is out there to support us.

- For instance, Jane mentioned that in some areas there are clinical pharmacists who might have more time to discuss medication. However, most of us had no idea that this role existed and might be available where we live.

- As George, our friend living with dementia, said: *'Psychosocial things like art, not just walking but exercise, being out in nature, gardening … doing things that we know are naturally good for people, that a lot of people don't have access to unless they are helped. Signposting is not enough. You have to hold a hand, take them to it, and get them started'*.

- Signposting is good – it is better to know than not know – but signposting is passive and it does not allow for individual circumstances. It would be better if GPs knew how to point you to the person who has the relevant information. This co-ordinator would know the full list of what was available in that area and be able to play matchmaker and signpost us to the **right** place. This could suit us because it is something we want, like an exercise class or a choir, something we can realistically attend, because it is served by public transport or allows someone living alone with dementia to attend by themselves, or something which fits our abilities – for example, directing someone in the mild stages of dementia to a memory café mainly attended by people with advanced dementia is unhelpful and upsetting. By the time we have been signposted to two things which do not suit us, we give up trying to seek help or support.

- Related to the previous point, policy-makers need to look across the country to ensure that there are things being provided everywhere, including more deprived areas and rural or less populated areas. We all deserve the opportunity to be directed to services and support which suit us rather than be told 'well, it's a postcode lottery' (and we lost).

- While we recognise the difficulties of information-sharing and personal data, it would be wonderful if healthcare professionals could share information so that we had proactive invitations from alternative local providers: community taxi services, activities, and more. It might require the input of policy-makers to enable this information-sharing: make decisions which shape systems to work better – many people will benefit.

- We need to have one consistent person to help us navigate the system. That single point of contact is invaluable – someone who knows us, our family, and our environment and understands what they need to pull in when. This would be so much more efficient than endlessly explaining the situation to a new person; by the time they have got the hang of it, something else has changed, so you are always fighting. We need a single point of contact who can be that liaison and co-ordinate the care needed.

- Be proactive rather than reactive: we should not need to get to crisis point. Offering crisis care or a crisis hotline is anything but reassuring – it tells us to expect crises. Highlight the services and support you offer which proactively keep us from crisis: that is reassuring. Dementia is going to throw enough little (and not-so-little) crises at us without the system doing it too.

> **10. We urge you: do something, change something, because every action makes a difference.**

Based on all our discussions and work on co-producing this book, this is our final manifesto point.

What you can do and the change you can effect will depend on your situation and your role. Policy-makers can change the way systems work for the better. Medics and other professionals can adopt ways of working which better suit us. Members of the public can learn about dementia, be understanding and patient when we take more time in front of you in the queue or warn community members about a potential scam on a local Facebook group. Although it is at different levels, everyone has the power to make change happen.

Dementia already affects an enormous number of people and is set to affect hundreds of thousands more. While drug discovery necessarily has an elongated timetable, social, attitudinal, environmental, and systemic changes need not wait. Now is the time to make a change.

Index

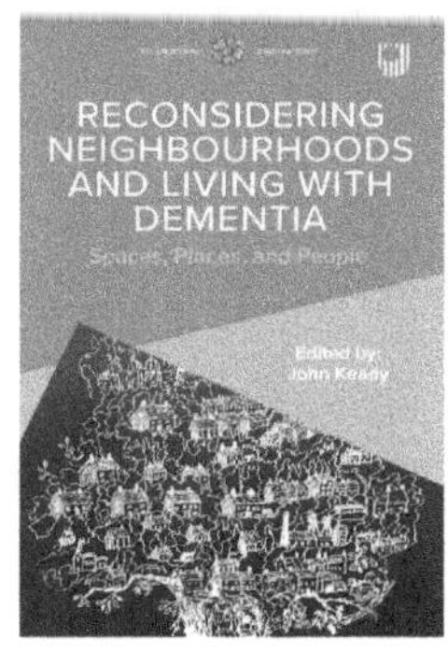

Reconsidering Neighbourhoods and Living with Dementia:
Spaces, Places and People

John Keady

ISBN: (Paperback) 9780335251728
eISBN: 9780335251735

2024

This book provides research based insights into the lived experience of dementia, aging in place and the use of participatory and creative social research approaches in the field of dementia studies. For the first time the key findings of one of the UKs largest funded social science research projects, the Neighbourhoods study, are assembled into one accessibly written blueprint for dementia care aiding better understanding of the place and position of those living with dementia in the home and neighbourhood context.

Reconsidering Neighbourhoods and Living with Dementia highlights the importance of home for people living with dementia and that neighbourhoods are seen to be relational, virtual, technological, connected, lived, remembered, and imagined, and to exist within and across time. The book is organised under **five key parts:**

- **The Lived Neighbourhood**
- **Neighbourhoods, Measurement and Technology**
- **Neighbourhoods and Big Data**
- **Personal Well-Being and Neighbourhood Programme Support**
- **Bringing it Together and Future Directions**

This comprehensive book is appropriate to a wide range of readers and disciplines including those living with dementia, the related health and voluntary professions, family carers, practitioners, academics, and students undertaking a variety of courses aligned to gerontology, dementia studies and human geography

www.mheducation.co.uk

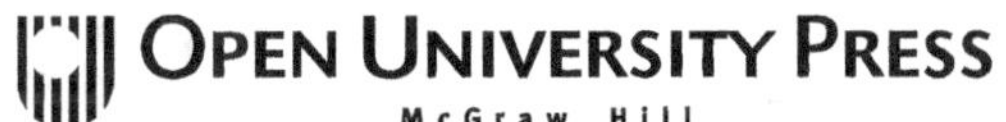

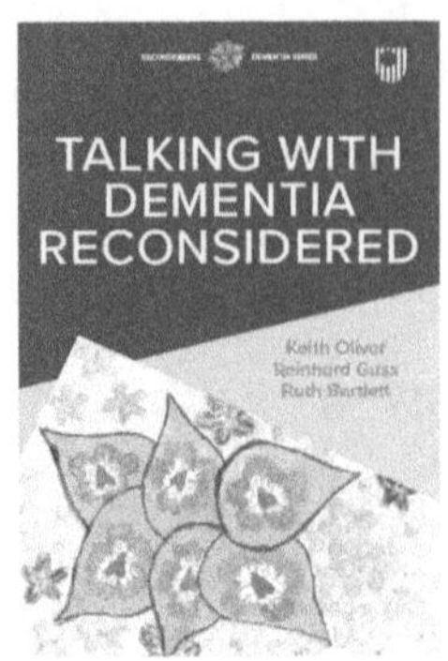

Talking with Dementia Reconsidered

Keith Oliver, Reinhard Guss, Ruth Bartlett

ISBN: 9780335251285 (Paperback)
eISBN: 9780335251292

2024

This book places people living with a diagnosis of dementia at its core, providing each person with the opportunity to express themselves whilst viewing their lives in relation to the Kitwood flower model.

Authored by a person living with dementia, an experienced consultant clinical psychologist and a respected academic, the three combine to amplify and showcase the words of the Fifteen people living with dementia in an original, authentic and unique way. This book:

- Gives readers transparent insight into the lives, hopes and fears of a diverse range of people living with various forms of dementia
- Shows how each petal of the Kitwood flower with love at its centre is a helpful framework for each person to describe their life
- Links the interviews with issues, frameworks, policy and practice
- Examines what stakeholders can take from this book to advance dementia care

Talking with Dementia Reconsidered truthfully adds to the growing knowledge base of what life with dementia is really like in an engaging and informative way. It is essential reading for anyone and everyone directly or indirectly affected by dementia through lived experience, studying dementia or working professionally to support those affected.

www.mheducation.co.uk

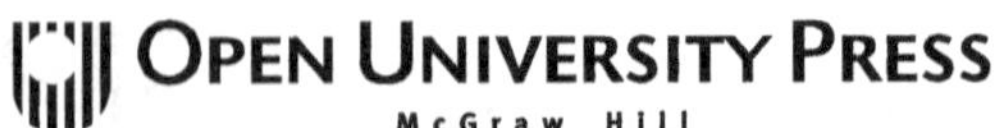

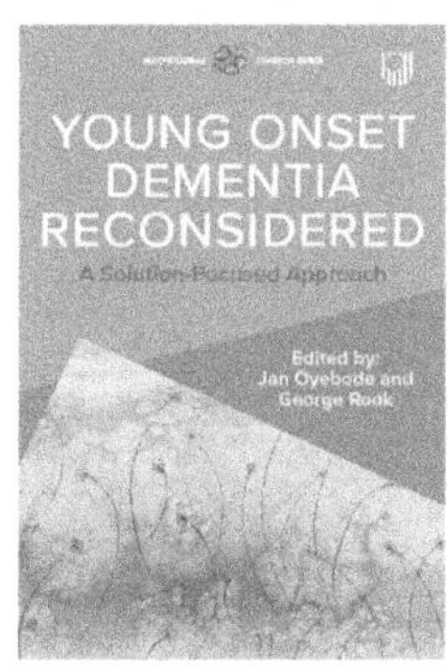

Young Onset Dementia Reconsidered:
A Solution Focused Approach

Jan Oyebode, George Rook

ISBN: 9780335252497 (Paperback)
eISBN: 9780335252503

2025

This solution-focused book, authored by leading experts from the UK, Canada, Norway and the Netherlands, delves into the many areas of life affected by dementia. When dementia occurs under 65 there are unique challenges and the impact on life is very different from diagnosis at a later age. The authors synthesise research to provide practical advice and information on living well, as well as the types of support available to those living with young onset dementia and their families.

Young Onset Dementia Reconsidered is accessibly written and split into three sections to reflect key outcomes important to people living with young onset dementia: to maintain control over their own lives, to retain a sense of identity and to feel connected with others. This book:

- Began from conversations with people living with young onset dementia and amplifies their voices throughout
- Contains coverage of a breadth of areas, including the social, psychological, employment, financial, legal and creative, as well as health and symptom-related aspects
- Is grounded in evidence and research and takes a solution-focused approach.

Jointly edited by one person living with young onset dementia and one clinical-academic with long experience of working in services, teaching and researching, *Young Onset Dementia Reconsidered* is a book for all those with an interest in dementia: students, practitioners, professionals, researchers, carers, family, friends and people with diagnosed or possible young onset dementia.

www.mheducation.co.uk

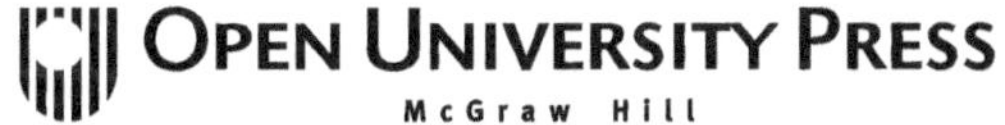